Cover illustration: 1882 New Zealand two pence postage stamp depicting Queen Victoria. The first synthetic dye, aniline purple or mauveine, was at first little known, but after the Queen wore a mauveine gown to the Great Exhibition of 1862, it became popular, and marked the beginning of the synthetic dye industry.

ii

MOLECULES, MADNESS, AND MALARIA

HOW VICTORIAN FABRIC DYES EVOLVED INTO MODERN MEDICINES FOR MENTAL ILLNESS AND INFECTIOUS DISEASE

Wallace B. Mendelson

Pythagoras Press

New York

About the author

Wallace B. Mendelson, MD is Professor of Psychiatry and Clinical Pharmacology (ret) at the University of Chicago. He is a Distinguished Fellow of the American Psychiatric Association and a member of the American Academy of Neuropsychopharmacology. He has been director of the Section on Sleep Studies at the National Institute of Mental Health, the Sleep Disorders Center at the Cleveland Clinic Foundation, and the Sleep Research Laboratory at the University of Chicago. He is the author of eight books and numerous professional papers. Among his honors have been the Academic Achievement Award from the American Sleep Disorders Association in 1999 and an award for excellence in sleep and psychiatry from the National Sleep Foundation in 2010. More information about Dr. Mendelson and his work is available on Wikipedia- https://en.wikipedia.org/wiki/Wallace_B._Mendelson and on his website- http://zhibit.org/wallacemendelson.

Disclaimer & Conflict of Interest Statement

CONFLICT OF INTEREST: Dr. Mendelson has no financial arrangements with any pharmaceutical company marketing any medicines mentioned in this book.

DISCLAIMER: This book contains information on a variety of medical and psychiatric disorders as well as their treatments. It is not a substitute for medical evaluation and treatment. If you believe you have any of the illnesses mentioned in this book, please consult your doctor.

Table of Contents

INTRODUCTION

My recent book *The Curious History of Medicines in Psychiatry* told the story of how in the 1950s and 1960s a number of creative individuals transformed often-accidental observations into the discoveries of new drugs.[1] By way of background, it touched upon how these were made possible by the burgeoning field of synthetic organic chemistry, and noted that it, too, began with a fortuitous discovery. In this case, William Henry Perkin, a chemistry student in London, was working with coal tar derivatives in 1856 and stumbled upon a darkly colored substance which became known as aniline purple dye. Thus began the synthetic dye industry, which branched out from textiles into other areas such as paints and cosmetics. After the success of aspirin in 1899, companies used their skills to develop medicines. In terms of psychiatry, this culminated a half century later in the clinical advent of chlorpromazine in 1952 and ushered in the modern era of psychopharmacology, in which new drugs grew often from serendipitous observations.

This new book comes from a growing realization that there is also another story to be told. It starts with Perkin's original goal; he was part of group at what became the Imperial College, and they were interested in the synthesis of quinine. In the nineteenth century, malaria was devastating the project of building and maintaining a worldwide empire, and there was great interest in preventing and treating it. In retrospect, this was a clue to the later history of drug development, in which it became clear that drugs for mental illness were not created in isolation. In fact, they grew hand in hand with the discoveries of antibacterials and antimalarials built from coal tar and derivative dyes, and interacted in a number of surprising ways. Perhaps the most famous of these was the discovery of chlorpromazine, a failed antimalarial, for psychoses.

It would have been difficult to tell this story of the complex relations between these two growing fields in a book about how inadvertent observations in post-World War II medicine were transformed into psychiatric drugs without losing a sense of narrative. Thus, the background of the previous book has become the foreground of this one, telling how in the century before chlorpromazine efforts to treat infectious diseases and psychiatric disorders grew from synthetic dyes, then developed and interacted together. In the 1930s, for instance, German pharmacologists, in a previously unsuccessful effort to develop azo dyes into antibacterial agents, used an old trick for making dyes adhere to fabrics by attaching a sulfonamide group; the result was Prontosil, the first sulfa drug. We will see how a penicillin preservative became the first modern tranquilizer, and how one trail to the precursor of the first antidepressants came from sulfa drugs. The benzodiazepine tranquilizers discovered in the 1950s were derived from previous work with unsatisfactory azo fabric dyes.

The back-and-forth in the evolution of antimicrobials and psychiatric medicines came to a close in the 1940s, as microbiologists moved from synthesis of dye-derived drugs such as Salvarsan and the sulfas to streptomycin, derived from soil bacteria, and penicillin, discovered from airborne mold. The two fields began to move off in their own directions. This book emphasizes an earlier period, and through a different lens—a wide-angle lens, if you will—telling the story of how efforts to treat infectious diseases and psychiatric disorders developed and interacted together. They were influenced by, and in turn affected, the world wars and the struggle to overcome the diseases of particular importance at that time: malaria, tuberculosis, and syphilis. It was an intriguing century-long process in which coal tar, a by-product of the industrial revolution, became the chemical building block for the evolution of new medicines. This, then, is the story of the growth of antibacterials and psychotropics, rambunctious siblings born of the dye industry and nourished by organic chemistry.

Just as it is useful to take a broader view of the context of these discoveries, it's worthwhile to look more widely at the background of the discoverers. It has been often noted that one of their important qualities was the willingness to accept unexpected observations and draw new implications from them. It's also easier to understand what they did by considering their backgrounds and predilections. August Kekulé had originally set out to be an architect and was a very visual person who sometimes had moments in which he saw molecules dancing; it is not so surprising that in 1865 his idea of a benzene ring involved a visual image of a structure, which he quickly sketched. Alexander Fleming's experiences in World War I produced a longstanding interest in finding natural substances to treat wounds, which served him well on the day in 1928 that he walked into the lab and found mold growing in one of his petri dishes. Similarly, Gerhard Domagk, who had tended wounds in field hospitals in the Great War, was likely to have had this on his mind when he developed sulfa antibacterials, and in the process saved his daughter's life from an infection. In the 1950s, when Leo Sternbach was tasked with finding novel kinds of molecules for tranquilizers (which became the benzodiazepines), he fell back on using as a starting point a group of dye compounds he had worked with in the 1930s as a student. This new book emphasizes that, in addition to chance events and a willingness to see things in the unexpected, past experiences and ways of thinking played a role in discoveries.

A few notes about the book itself: This is a free-standing project, and so of necessity touches on some of the topics from *The Curious History of Medicines in Psychiatry*. This includes the Prologue, which describes the origins of organic chemistry, and Chapter Two, which summarizes the discoveries in psychiatry in the 1950s. They are told from a different perspective, however. The section on chlorpromazine, for instance, is entitled 'How a failed antimalarial revolutionized psychiatry' and emphasizes how its ancestral dyes, and the new drug itself, were enlisted in the struggle against this global disease. The history of isoniazid, the precursor to the first MAO inhibitor antidepressant, is broadened: instead of describing its traditional origin in the U.S. as a derivative of rocket fuel, it is shown to have also come in the same year from a European laboratory which created it from sulfa antibacterials. The hope is that viewing it in this way will emphasize that the growth of medicines in psychiatry did not happen in isolation, but rather was part of a dynamic process involving other types of medicines and disorders.

Finally, I have tried to write this in a manner that is available to readers with a wide range of backgrounds, with a goal that it will be useful and enjoyable for anyone with an interest in how drugs came to be discovered. In a few cases where it seemed important, there are footnotes and references for the more technically minded reader. These are minimal, though, in the interest of telling a free-flowing story of how the struggle against diseases in the setting of world events and new technologies, and some remarkable individuals, helped make the world as it is today.

PROLOGUE: SYNTHETIC ORGANIC CHEMISTRY

A student's spring break project opened a new field of chemistry.

L
ong before the days of 'chemistry sets,' modern organic chemistry was launched by a student's accident with a smelly chemical while experimenting in his attic. William Henry Perkin (1838-1907) was a precocious young scholar at London Day School when one of his teachers convinced his father that rather than pursuing architecture, he should follow a career in chemistry. In 1853, the 15-year-old Perkin enrolled in the Royal College of Chemistry (later part of Imperial College, London). At that time the director was a famous German chemist named August Wilhelm von Hofmann (1818-1892), who believed that coal tar, essentially an industrial waste product produced in making coal gas, could be used to make alkaloids, plant-based organic compounds usually containing nitrogen atoms, which had many uses including as medicines. This was during the time of the Crimean War, in which British soldiers suffered from a variety of infectious diseases such as typhus, cholera, and malaria. The only available treatment for malaria in those days was the alkaloid

quinine, derived from the bark of the South American and Polynesian cinchona tree, and incidentally the substance which gives the characteristic taste to tonic water. (For the history of quinine, see Chapter Three). Von Hofmann suggested to Perkin that he try to find a way to synthesize quinine.

Though Perkin was busy with other projects at the College, he built a laboratory in the attic of his house in East London. In a way this was a chancy thing to do—not long before, one of his fellow students had burned to death while attempting to derive benzene from coal tar. During Easter vacation in 1856, he attempted to form quinine by adding oxygen atoms to a complex coal tar derivative, but sadly he only produced a brown mess in his equipment*. He then decided to work with a simpler molecule known as aniline, an oily, colorless liquid redolent of spoiled fish. Attempting to combine it with potassium dichromate, an orange-red powder, he dissolved both in hot water and then mixed them together. This time he was rewarded, not with quinine, but with a black sticky substance. In an effort to remove it from his glassware, he added alcohol, and was surprised to see that it formed a liquid with a rich purple color, which adhered to the cleaning cloth.

---

* To be more precise, his goal was oxidizing the complex amine allyltoluidine, and then in a second study aniline, with potassium dichromate. It seems likely that he was using impure aniline, and the resultant aniline purple dye, after extracting with alcohol, was a mixture of several molecules.

As it happened, Perkin was very sensitive to color, perhaps due to his longstanding interest in photography and painting, and it occurred to him that his newfound substance might be useful as a dye for fabrics. At the time, purple dye was largely derived at great expense from the mucous secretion of mollusks and, because of its scarcity, was associated with wealth and royalty. Perkin raised the possibility that it could be mass-produced at low cost. He presented the idea to Hofmann, who initially dismissed it as trivial and urged him to focus on quinine. Perkin felt otherwise and, along with his brother and a friend, built a laboratory to pursue his interest in what he called aniline purple. After applying it to silk himself and then a successful test in a silk dye works in Scotland, he patented it in 1856 and founded a company without much success at first. Eventually its vivid look and colorfastness in silk caught the royal eye; after it was favored by the French Empress Eugénie and was worn by Queen Victoria at the Royal Exhibition of 1862, its popularity soared, appearing not only in clothes but also in British 'penny lilac' postage stamps.

EXPOSITION UNIVERSELLE DE 1862.

Suite. — Voy. p. 205, 235, 273.

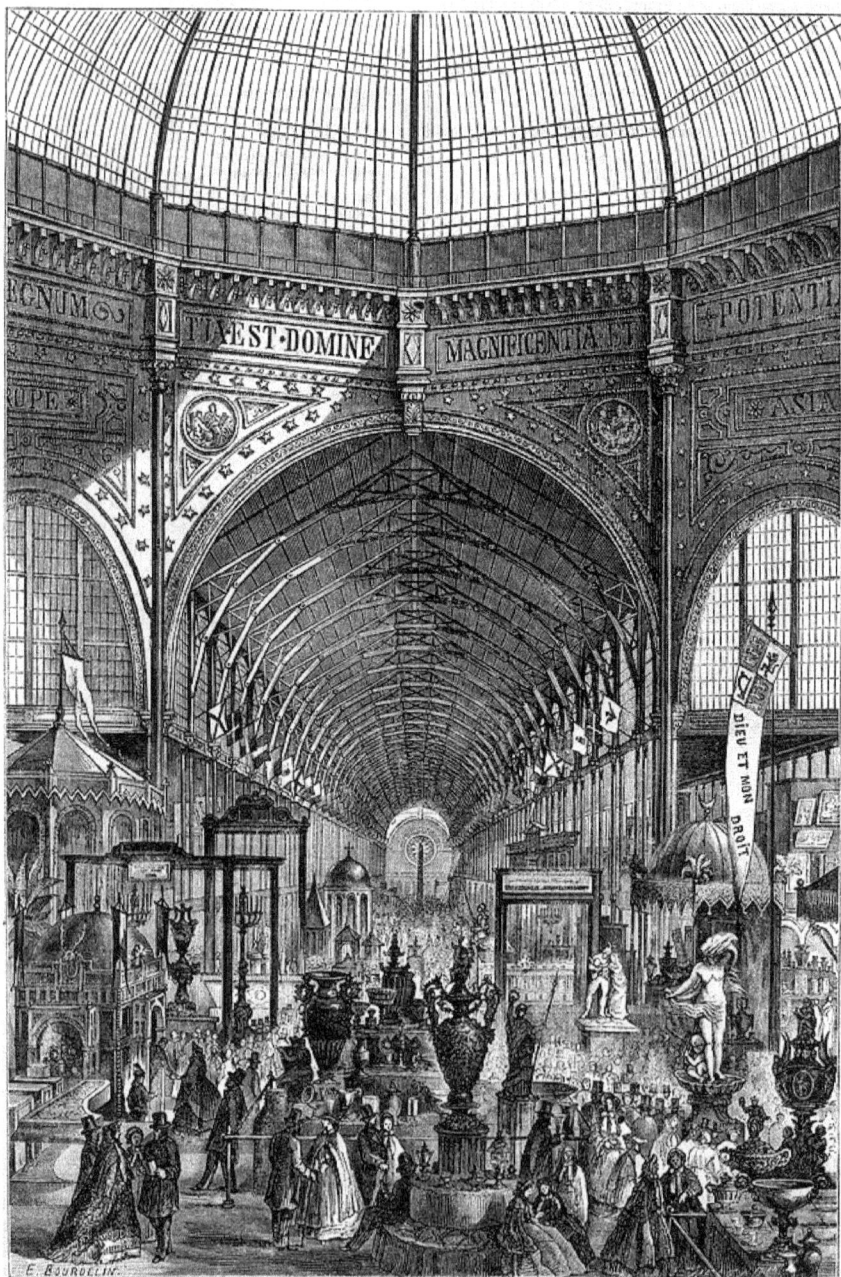

Exposition universelle de Londres en 1862; vue intérieure. — Dessin de Bourdelin.

11

Figure P-1: The Great Exhibition of 1862 was a world's fair in London, bringing together exhibitors from 36 countries. The displays included Charles Babbage's analytical engine (a mechanical computer), undersea cables, and the electric telegraph. Queen Victoria's gown, colored with Perkin's aniline purple, spurred public interest in the new dye.

Perkin's success with the dye, which came to be known by the French names mauve or mauveine (for the mallow flower of a similar color), led the founding of a number of dye companies, which with expanded interests still exist today, including Bayer, Ciba, Geigy, and Sandoz. Though Perkin never synthesized quinine—that was not to happen until 1944 (see Chapter Three)—he had opened up the field of synthetic organic chemistry. As we will see later, the early dye companies used their newly developed skills to expand into other areas, including paints, cosmetics, food coloring, and—most importantly for our discussion—medicines.

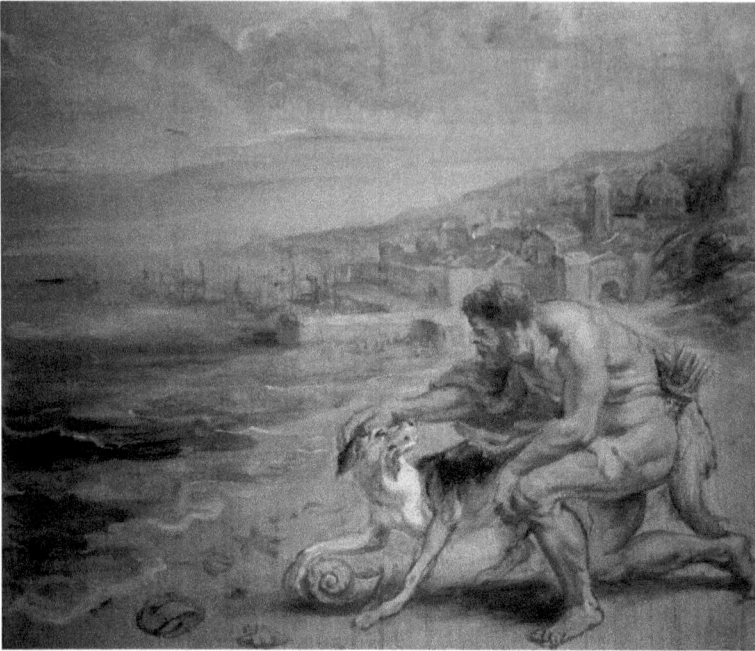

Figure P-2: Hercules and the discovery of the secret of purple. In this 1636 painting, the Flemish Peter Paul Rubens (1577-1640) illustrates the legend of how Tyrian purple was discovered. Hercules was on his way to an amorous visit with the nymph Tyro when his dog found and bit into a sea snail, a type of mollusk (depicted, with artistic freedom by Rubens, as a nautilus). The unfortunate creature's fluids stained the dog's mouth purple. Tyro thought the color would be just the thing for a new gown, which began the practice of using Tyrian purple as a fabric dye. The Phoenicians in the second millennium BC wore it, and one theory holds that the word 'Phoenicia' comes from 'land of purple.' In ancient times, it was worn by Greek senators and Roman Generals. In Perkin's day, it continued to convey a sense of rank and wealth. As a result of his discovery of synthetic aniline purple dye, purple fabrics ultimately came into widespread use.

Before all this could happen, though, one more hurdle had to be overcome. When the 18-year-old Perkin was stumbling upon aniline purple, the state of chemistry was such that it was possible to determine the composition of organic compounds, but the structure formed when carbon and other atoms were connected was unknown. In 1858, another architect/chemist, August Kekulé, and Archibald Scott Couper found the answer.

August Kekulé, Archibald Scott Couper, and carbon-based structures

August Kekulé (1829-1896), the son of a civil servant in Darmstadt in southern Germany, showed an aptitude for drawing and ultimately was encouraged by his parents to study architecture at the University of Giessen. There he fell under the spell of Justus Liebig, a chemist and popular lecturer who previously in 1832 had made chloral hydrate, which went on some years later to become the first synthetic drug for sleep. Switching to chemistry with his family's support, he ultimately obtained a doctorate in 1852, but was unable to find an academic position. After postdoctoral work in Switzerland and England, he went to Heidelberg, where he built his own laboratory in a corn merchant's house (reminiscent of William Henry Perkin's attic laboratory) and became a *Privatdozent* (an unpaid teacher) at the University of Heidelberg from 1855 to 1858. He was very interested in carbon atoms and how they might bind to other atoms. He began to develop a theory, which in retrospect he said had come to him from a daydream of dancing molecules while atop a double-decker horse-drawn bus in London in 1855. In 1858, he published a groundbreaking paper in which he proposed that carbon was tetravalent, that is, was capable of attaching to as many as four other atoms and could link together with other carbon atoms to form chains and other shapes. His career blossomed; at the age of 29 he was asked to be the chairman of the chemistry department at the University of Ghent, and later took a similar role at the University of Bonn, where he reigned as the most famous chemist of his age.

As it turned out, Kekulé was not alone in his reasoning. Archibald Scott Couper (1831-1892), a Scottish chemist working in Paris, came out with similar ideas in the same year. He gave a paper outlining his notions to his chairman, Charles-Adolphe Wurtz, famous for his work on organic compounds of nitrogen and ammonia, for submission to the French Academy. Wurtz apparently was delayed in his submission, and ultimately Couper's paper was published two months after Kekulé's. Couper, very upset, quarreled with his boss and was fired. Though he was offered a position in Edinburgh, he was so distraught that he ultimately was psychiatrically hospitalized and was never able to resume his profession.

One mystery which remained after Kekulé and Couper's success was how to picture the structure of compounds such as benzene, previously discovered in 1825, which was comprised of exactly six carbon and six hydrogen atoms. Kekulé later realized that the carbon atoms must be joined together in a ring. As he described it retrospectively, one evening in 1865, he was having difficulty writing a particular passage, turned toward the fireplace, and 'fell half asleep.' He then once again had a vision of dancing atoms connected in rows and writhing like snakes. One of the snakes bit its own tail, forming a circle. Awakening, Kekulé realized he was on to something, and worked the rest of the night, developing the notion of the ring structure of carbon atoms making up the molecule of benzene. This opened up the study of aromatic organic chemistry (focusing on compounds which include a carbon ring structure), representing the majority of organic molecules, that is, molecules comprised of carbon, hydrogen, oxygen, and other atoms). This greatly boosted the chemical industry, which could now work not only with the constituent atoms of substances, but how they came together to build structures. As time went on, it became clear that carbon atoms could link together not only in chains and rings, but in complex shapes including tubes and spheres. Organic substances comprise the majority of types of molecules, and indeed carbon-based molecules are more common than the sum total of those from other elements. Thus, they provided a rich field to develop dyes, paints, cosmetics, agricultural chemicals, explosives, plastics—and medicines.

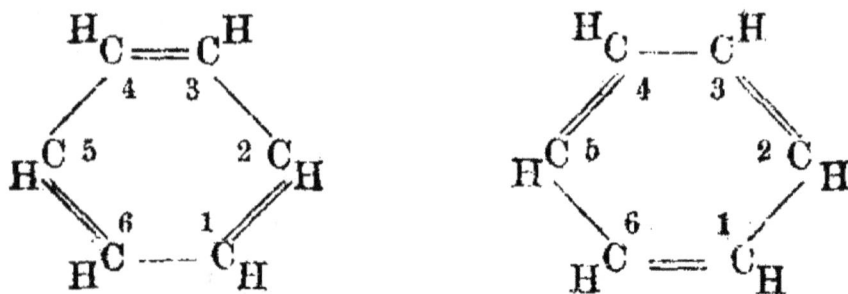

Figure P-3: Kekulé's drawing of the structure of benzene*. In this 1872 version, he suggests that the ring moves back and forth into two equivalent structures, in which the single and double bonds alternate their positions constantly.

Adolph von Bayer's discovery of barbiturates: Around the time of Kekulé's formulation of the benzene ring, one of his chemists made a groundbreaking discovery in the history of sedative medicines. Adolph von Bayer (1835-1917) had been a student of Robert Bunsen (as in the 'Bunsen burner') but quarreled with him and instead studied with Kekulé in Germany. After

---

* He described it as follows: "[...] you can see, therefore, that each carbon atom collides with the other two with which it collides with the same number of times, i.e., it has exactly the same relationship with its two neighbors. The usual benzene formula, of course, only expresses the bursts occurring in one unit of time [...], and so one has been led to believe that biderivatives with the positions 1,2 and 1,6 should necessarily be different. If the idea just shared or a similar one can be considered correct, it follows that this difference is only an apparent one, but not a real one." Translated from: August Kekulé (1872). "Ueber einige Condensationsproducte des Aldehyds". *Liebigs Ann. Chem.* **162** (1): 77–124. DOI:10.1002/jlac.18721620110

receiving his doctorate, von Bayer moved with him to Ghent, where Kekulé charged him with the task of making a cyclic ring molecule out of the seemingly ill-matched combination of urea (a constituent of urine) and malonic acid (found in apples). He succeeded one night and decided to celebrate his achievement at a nearby tavern. When he arrived, however, there was already a party in progress. Soldiers from a nearby barracks were celebrating the special day of Saint Barbara, the patron saint of the artillery. The legend goes that somehow during the festivities, an alcohol-fueled inspiration led to combining the word 'urea' with Saint Barbara, resulting in the name 'barbiturate' for the new compound. Variations on this story involve a barmaid named Barbara who may have contributed specimens for urea, as well as a derivation from the German word *Schlusselbart*, referring to the bit of a key, as von Bayer viewed it as the key to a wide range of compounds. In any event, over the years, perhaps 2,500 different barbiturate compounds were developed, resulting in about 50 medicines.

As it happens, barbituric acid, the compound created by von Bayer, is not psychoactive. It was not until 1903 that one of his former students, Emil Fischer, and the German physician Joseph von Mering, modified the molecule to produce the first barbiturate sedative, barbital (Veronal). In the ensuing years, related compounds were developed as anesthetics, anticonvulsants, tranquilizers, and sleeping pills. They remained the dominant sedatives until the advent of the benzodiazepines ('Valium-like' drugs) in the 1960s. As for von Bayer himself, he went on to synthesize indigo dye with his colleague Heinrich Caro, as well as fluorescent dyes, and a precursor to what would become one of the first plastics. He was awarded the Nobel Prize in 1905, as had Fisher in 1901 and von Mering in 1902.

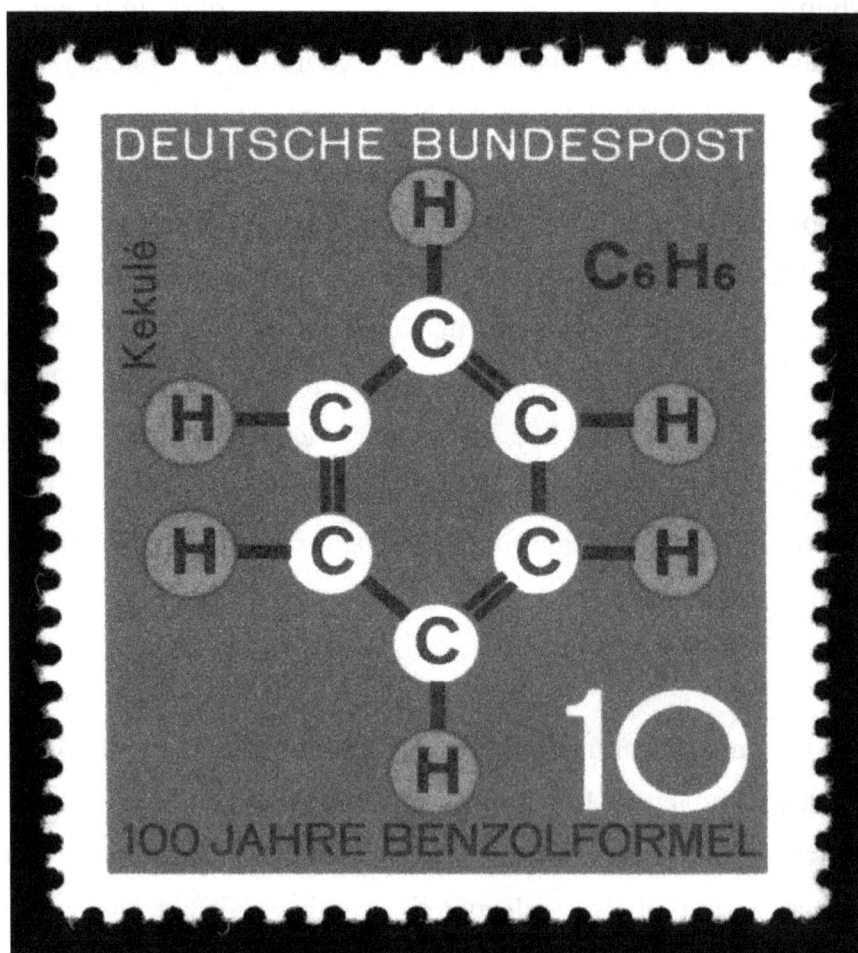

Figure P-4: *A West German 1964 stamp commemorating centenary of the discovery of the structure of benzene.*

Discoveries that come while sleeping: In passing, it's interesting that Kekulé's dream image of a snake biting its tail was also a symbol going back to the ancient Egyptians, known as an *ouroboros*, used by the classical Greeks and later becoming an emblem of alchemy. Kekulé, like William Henry Perkin, was a very visual person, interested at an early age in art and a budding architect who became a chemist. The idea of structures, how things were put together, was very important to him, just as color was important to Perkin. They both bring to mind the story of Ramon y Cajal (1852-1934), their Spanish contemporary, who wanted to become an artist but followed his father's urgings to become a physician and ultimately won acclaim for his drawings of nerve cells in the structure of the brain (see the companion book *Understanding Antidepressants*). Nor was Kekulé alone in having visual ideas during daydreams. The German physiologist Otto Loewi (1873-1961) awakened one night in 1921 with an idea for a crucial experiment and hastily scribbled down notes about it. The next morning, however, he was unable to read his nocturnal handwriting. The following night, he awakened with the same thought, but this time he hastened to his laboratory, where he conducted the crucial experiment which demonstrated chemical neurotransmission—the idea that nerve cells communicate by releasing chemicals which travel across a gap to signal the receiving neuron—for which he won the Nobel Prize.

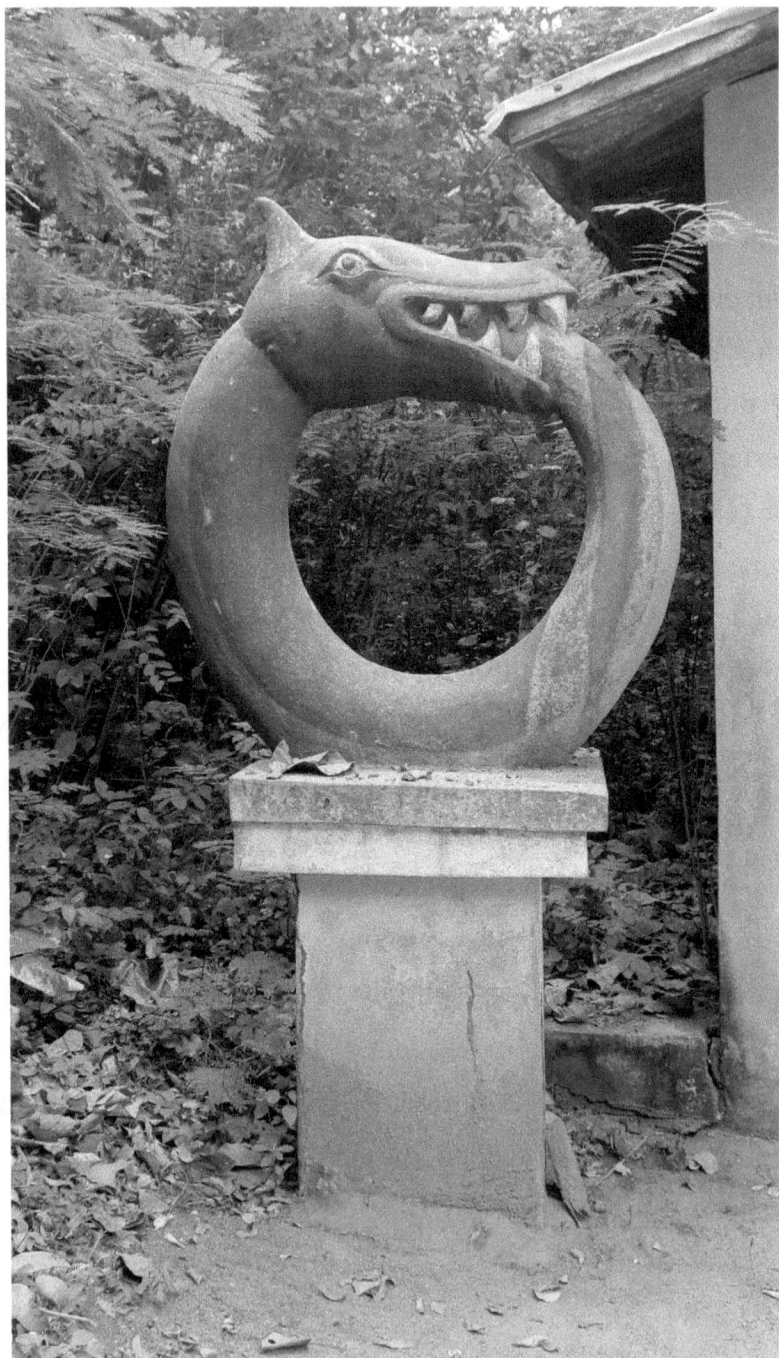

Figure P-5: Ouroboros statue in the Sacred Forest Ouidah Benin, January 2018.

CHAPTER ONE: DYES AND DRUGS

When Perkin and his successors began synthesizing a wide variety of useful products, they needed to have a starting material, rich in organic molecules, abundant, and inexpensive. As it happens, they had such a material readily available, in the form of coal tar. Let's take a brief look at how this came about, and then we'll describe some of the dyes and drugs that were derived from it.

The building block: Coal tar

Prior to the Industrial Revolution, whale oil had been a major source of lighting, as well as an ingredient in making soaps and lubricants. Surprisingly, it was a constituent of automatic transmission fluid in cars until banned in the U.S. in 1973. In practice, though, whaling began its decline in the nineteenth century, as coal gas became more popular.

Coal gas was piped into homes from large industrial facilities and remained a dominant form of lighting and heat until the 1940s and 1950s in the U.S., and a decade or two later in the U.K. (As an aside, it was also used in famous balloon flights, as portrayed in the movie *The Aeronauts**.) It was made by heating coal in the absence of oxygen, in the process of making coke for use in the iron industry. Originally considered a by-product, it became clear that it and other resultant materials including coal tar, ammonia, and sulfur had their own uses. Coal tar itself is a mixture of perhaps 10,000 different kinds of molecules, many of which are still not understood. It is a dark, oily liquid, which when distilled produces a variety of substances including tar for road surfacing, the wood preservative creosote, over-the-counter skin creams and shampoos for itching and scaling still used today, as well as phenols and other chemicals which became a rich source of raw materials for organic chemists. As coal tar was cheap and readily available, huge gasworks plants become a prominent feature of urban landscapes. It remained the major source material for dyes (as well as other products such as saccharin, paint, food coloring, and even explosives) until it was gradually replaced by petroleum derivatives in the last few decades. In the next sections, we will look at some of the dyes and, ultimately, medicines that were made from it.

---

* Released in 2019, the adventure film starring Felicity Jones and Eddie Redmayne was based on Richard Holmes' 2013 book *How we Took to the Air*, and depicts a fictionalized version of a record-breaking flight of a coal gas balloon in 1862.

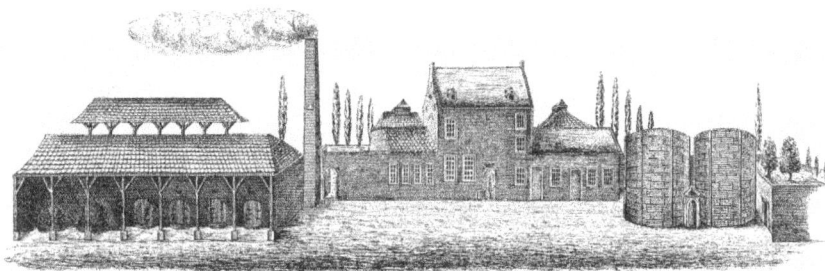

Figure 1-1: Gasworks, in which coal gas was generated from heating coal in the absence of oxygen, began appearing in Europe around the beginning of the nineteenth century. They were often near the docks and later railways, often in the poorer parts of town. Youths from these areas were often called the 'gas house gang,' a name adopted by the St. Louis Cardinals in 1934. Ultimately with the advent of natural gas, gasworks were no longer needed, but the sites of many are still used as storage facilities. One of the byproducts of making natural gas was coal tar, which nineteenth century chemists recognized as a rich source of organic molecules that could be used as starting points for making new substances. This particular drawing was made of a gasworks built in Maastricht, The Netherlands, in 1847.

Methylene blue: The 'blue wonder' that became the first fully synthetic medicine

Methylene blue (MB), an azo dye related to aniline compounds, was first developed as a fabric dye in 1876 by Heinrich Caro, a German calico printer and chemist who later was the co-discoverer of the synthesis of indigo. There it might have remained, were it not for the work of Paul Ehrlich (1854-1915), one of the most remarkable figures in the history of pharmacology. Born in Silesia (now part of Poland), the son of an innkeeper and liquor distiller, he was heavily influenced by his older cousin Karl Weigert, a pathologist who was a pioneer in using aniline dyes to stain tissues for microscopy. After his medical training, Ehrlich continued this work, among other things using dyes to differentiate the main types of white blood cells. He became interested in using methylene blue for bacteria, just as his friend Robert Koch did in identifying the bacterium causing tuberculosis. Ehrlich also found that MB would stain axons (the long extensions by which nerve cells communicate).

In the process of his work at a tuberculosis unit in Berlin, he contracted the disease in 1888 and took two years off, traveling to Egypt and other places. During this period, he continued his work with methylene blue on his own and found that it stained the single-celled *Plasmodium* parasites responsible for malaria when transmitted by an infected *Anopheles* mosquito. In 1891, he and the pathologist Paul Guttmann recognized that it also was toxic to the *Plasmodium*, and they began to wonder whether it might be useful in the treatment of malaria. Indeed, when it was given to two patients in Berlin, they became better and the *Plasmodium* was no longer evident in their bloodstreams. In this leap from the microscope to the bedside, Ehrlich began to think of dyes as therapeutic agents, which could selectively stain the cell walls of bacteria and kill them or prevent their growth, and he viewed this as a new therapeutic approach. Indeed, many modern antibiotics such as penicillin work by altering the function of bacterial cell walls, so in a general sense he was correct, though there was much more to be learned.

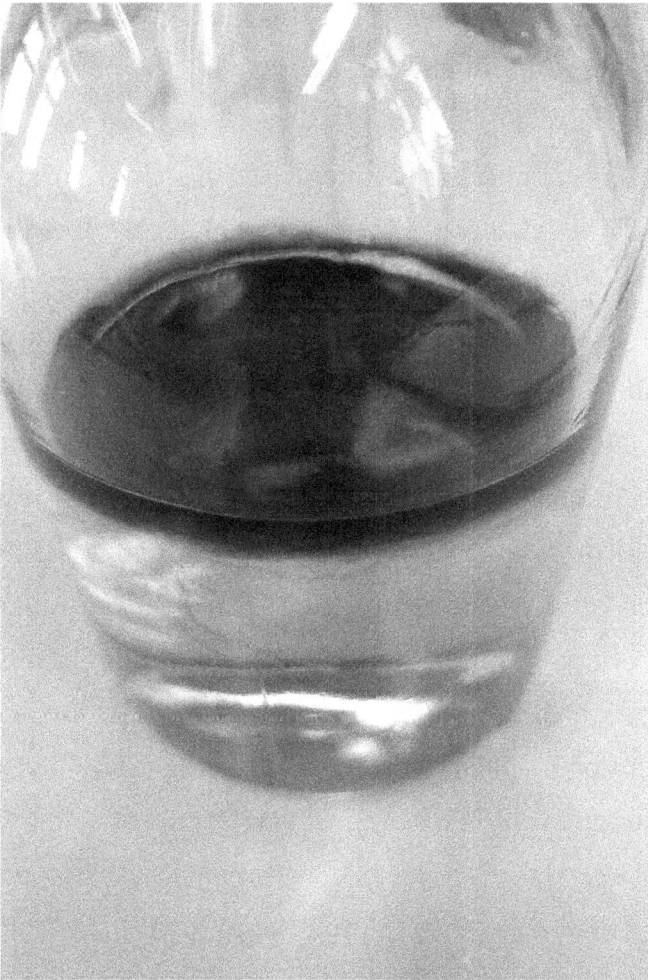

Figure 1-2: Methylene blue in ethanol. First discovered in 1876 as a fabric dye, it was used as an antimalarial and formed the basic building block of other drugs,

including chlorpromazine. Today it is still used to treat the illness methemoglobinemia and is being explored for a possible role in slowing the progression of Alzheimer's disease (Chapter Five).

In looking back over Ehrlich's career, the idea of dyes becoming therapy can be seen to have grown from a number of observations. In 1904, he and colleague Kiyoshi Shiga reported that the arsenical dye trypan red inhibited trypanosomes, the parasites causing sleeping sickness (Trypanosomiasis), and indeed he published a report on its benefits as a treatment. Atoxyl stain was developed by others as a drug for sleeping sickness but later became the starting point from which he ultimately developed Salvarsan for syphilis. He found that flavine yellow dye was lethal to bacteria in abscesses, and it went on to be an antiseptic used for wounds in World War I. Although it is arguable, there is less of a sense of there being a single dramatic 'Aha' moment, similar to when Frank Berger noticed that a penicillin preservative he was testing made animals docile and was struck by the idea that it might be a useful tranquilizer in humans (Chapter Three). Rather, Ehrlich's intuition came from the cumulative weight of a number of observations. He later developed the concept of 'magic bullets' in which dyes or other agents which bind to bacteria could be paired with a toxic substance which, once delivered, would selectively kill the desired target. His ideas were so pervasive that the words 'drug' and 'dye' were often used interchangeably as recently as World War I. Though the conclusion seemed inescapable, it's interesting that in a sense it was serendipitous—he had set out to learn how to visualize tissues and bacteria but reacted to unexpected observations with the intuitive leap that they could in fact become medical treatments.

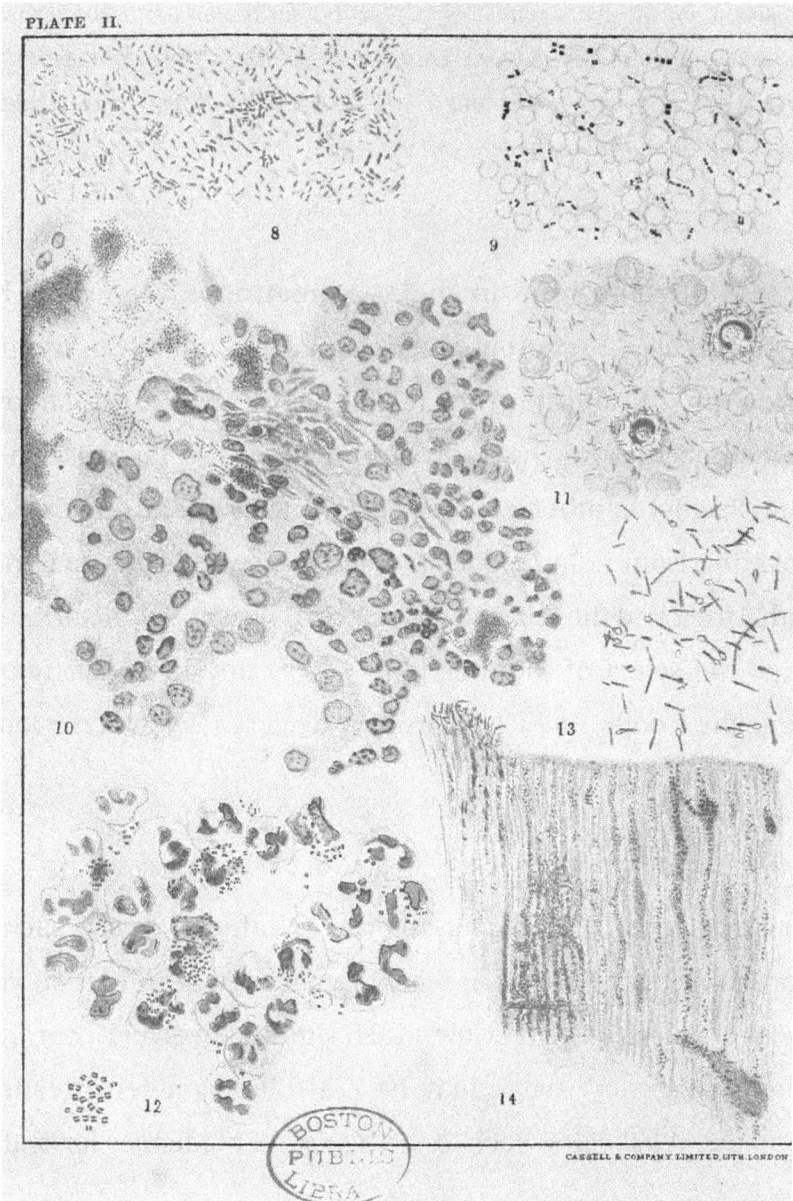

PLATE II.

Figure 1-3: Microscopic images of bacteria, from a surgical textbook of 1895. The sections 8 and 11 used methylene blue staining to show a culture of Bacillus Coli Communis and unspecified bacteria in the blood respectively. Around this time, Paul Ehrlich and colleague Paul Guttmann used methylene blue to stain the microscopic Plasmodium parasites responsible for malaria and noted that the stain itself seemed to inhibit them. This and observations with other stains led to Ehrlich's evolving idea that stains could be used as drugs to selectively kill bacteria without harming the infected person.

Methylene blue in malaria treatment: Methylene blue was indeed used to prevent and treat malaria, notably in troops in World Wars I and II. General Douglas MacArthur famously commented that for every division fighting the Japanese in the South Pacific, another was sick from malaria, and another was recovering from it. Indeed, 60,000 soldiers were lost to malaria in North Africa and the South Pacific. As MB discolored the urine and turned the sclera of the eyes blue, it was not a popular remedy among the troops, and a famous ditty declared 'Even at the loo we see, we pee, navy blue.'

Though largely replaced by newer synthetic drugs such as chloroquine, there has been recent renewed interest in methylene blue for malaria. One review of 21 studies involving over 1,000 patients suggested that it may have a role in modern treatment regimens[2]. We'll come back to the history of medicines for malaria in more detail in Chapter Three. The many other contemporary medical uses of methylene blue will be presented in Chapter Five.

Methylene blue in psychiatry: Because it produces blue-colored urine, MB was also given to psychiatric patients along with their regular treatments as a way to check whether they were taking their medicines. In this and other situations, it was observed that it might have antidepressant or sedative effects, which were noted by Ehrlich and other groups at the time[3]. Ehrlich predicted that it might be useful in psychiatric treatments but did not pursue this actively. As we will see in Chapter Two, he was prescient, as 50 years later, chlorpromazine, a methylene blue derivative which was unsuccessfully tested for antimalarial activity, became the first modern antipsychotic and revolutionized modern psychiatric treatment. We will see more of Ehrlich's heritage in the discussion of the discovery of Salvarsan for syphilis, later in this chapter.

Anti-fever drugs

In telling the story of methylene blue and its use in malaria, we jumped ahead to the development of the related compounds such as chloroquine in the twentieth century, and even to a renewed interest in methylene blue itself in the twenty-first. Let's return now to the years in the late nineteenth century in which methylene blue and other coal tar derivatives were being developed as dyes. One important step in those years was the synthesis by Kekulé's former student Adolph von Bayer and Heinrich Caro of indigo dye (now known for its coloration of blue jeans) in 1880, which after commercialization brought an end to the lucrative trade of plant-based indigo from India. (In Chapter Five, we will see how currently indigo derivatives are being developed as 'photoswitches' for potential use with infections and cancer.) But in those years, the coal tar derivative which led the way to the development of medicines was the discovery of acetylsalicylic acid, or aspirin.

Antipyrine: Although malaria was characterized by intermittent fevers, there are of course a host of illnesses that result in raised body temperature, and there was great interest in finding fever-reducing ('antipyretic') medicines. Technological advances such as the advent of the clinical thermometer in 1870 standardized and spurred their development as well. An early one was antipyrine, which came from the quinine derivate quinoline. Its presentation to the public followed the invention of the rotary tablet press in 1872, which paved the way for the widespread distribution of commercial drugs, and by 1883 antipyrine in an early form of a modern pill was being manufactured. Inevitably, it was soon replaced by aspirin, related to a compound in plants but ultimately synthesized as a coal tar derivative.

Aspirin: Willow bark as a medicine has its roots in ancient Sumer and Egypt. It was used extensively by the classical Greeks and

Romans, continuing into the Middle Ages and beyond. There was a surge of interest in it during the eighteenth century, when a Church of England chaplain, Edward Stone (1702-1768) took a walk near Chipping Norton, wishing he could get relief from his 'ague,' an ill-defined cluster of symptoms including fever, fatigue, and aches, which probably included malaria and other conditions.

Stone was a believer in the 'doctrine of signatures,' a now discredited view that herbs which resembled human body parts often contained cures for that part's ailments. In a more religious phrasing, it was thought that by shaping therapeutic plants to resemble the body, God was giving people a hint that help lies within. Thus, herbalists would use extracts of the liverwort plant to help liver disorders, or eyebright for infections of the eyes. In broader terms, it suggested that the cure of a malady lies close to its source. Since ague was thought to be contracted near swampy areas, he got the idea of nibbling on the bark of a willow tree growing by a marsh. At the time, he noticed a bitter flavor, which to him seemed similar to that of the Peruvian cinchona, which he had sampled in the past. He was happy to see that his symptoms improved, though the connection with malaria was unclear: as we have seen, the bitter-tasting active ingredient in cinchona bark which kills malaria parasites is quinine, while the willow's active ingredient, salicylic acid, merely provides some relief from the fever and aches which accompany it and other conditions. Stone tested a powder made from the willow on around 50 others, then wrote an enthusiastic letter to the Royal Society in 1763.

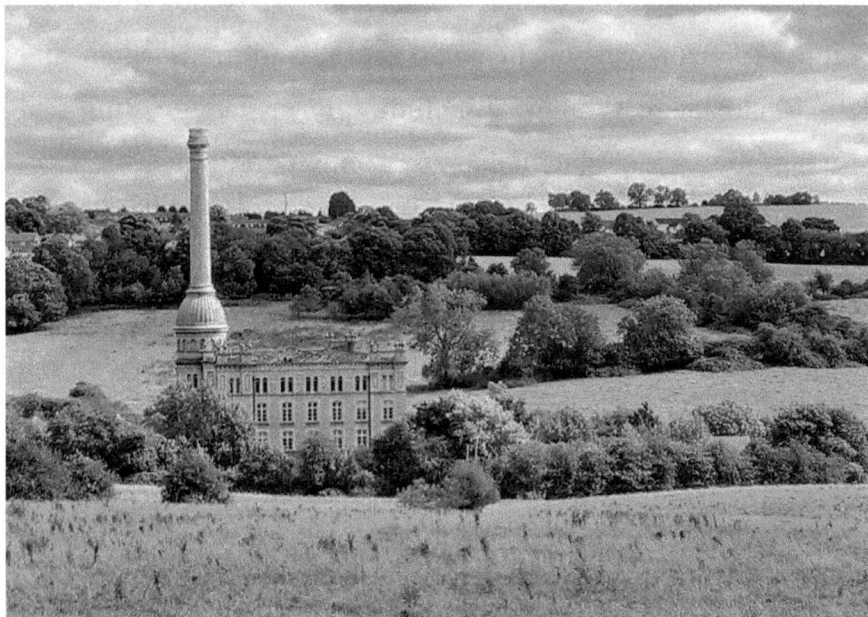

Figure 1-4: Chipping Norton, a small market town in Oxfordshire, England, and historically a center of the wool trade in the Cotswold Hills, in this 2014 photo. Reverend Stone strolled the nearby meadows in 1763 and decided to sample the willow bark. The mill would have not been there in his time; it was built in 1872 to manufacture tweed cloth from wool.

Studies of the active substance in willow bark were stirred in the early nineteenth century as a consequence of the Napoleonic wars and shipping blockades. By the 1820s, it was recognized that the active ingredient was salicin (from the Latin for 'willow'), or salicylic acid. In 1853, the Alsatian chemist Charles Frédéric Gerhardt produced acetylsalicylic acid from sodium salicylate, but the structure was unknown and the synthesis awkward. Over the course of the next half century, both of these limitations were overcome. In the late nineteenth century, the complete synthesis of acetylsalicylic acid was worked out, starting with the coal tar derivatives benzene and phenol. (Phenol itself had been synthesized by Kekulé and Charles-Adolphe Wurtz, who we mentioned in the Prologue was Archibald Scott Couper's director, in 1867.) In 1899, the Bayer company marketed acetylsalicylic acid as Aspirin (the 'a' coming from 'acetyl,' while the 'spir' was derived from *Spirea ulmaria*, the Meadowsweet plant, one source of salicylic acid).

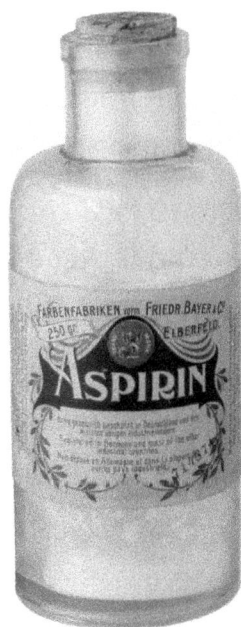

Figure 1-5: An 1899 bottle of aspirin.

Aspirin's popularity was, to use a current phrase, viral, and it soon came to be recognized as an important medicine coming from Bayer's German and German-controlled American factories. With the advent of World War I, however, phenol production was diverted for use in the explosive trinitrophenol*, and Great Britain's naval embargo reduced supplies further. In what became known as 'the great phenol plot,' German spies, among them an ex-Bayer employee, arranged to buy phenol from Thomas Edison, who needed it for producing vinyl records and indeed had built his own factory to make it. Though Edison did, possibly unknowingly, sell them phenol for some time, the plot ultimately was foiled when the Secret Service discovered incriminating documents after one of the conspirators accidentally left his briefcase on a train, and the supply for Germany was cut off. After the war, demand for aspirin continued to rise, and to this day it represents one of the most widely used medicines in the world. Another phenol-derived pain medicine, acetaminophen (Panadol, Tylenol, and other brands), first synthesized in 1877 but marketed in the U.S. since the 1950s, remains popular as well. Phenol itself now largely comes from petroleum rather than coal tar.

---

* Trinitrophenol was a more powerful explosive, though less stable than TNT (trinitrotoluene). One reason for its widespread use was that toluene, also derived from coal tar and other sources, was in shorter supply, but TNT-based munitions gradually replaced trinitrophenol because of relatively greater safety.

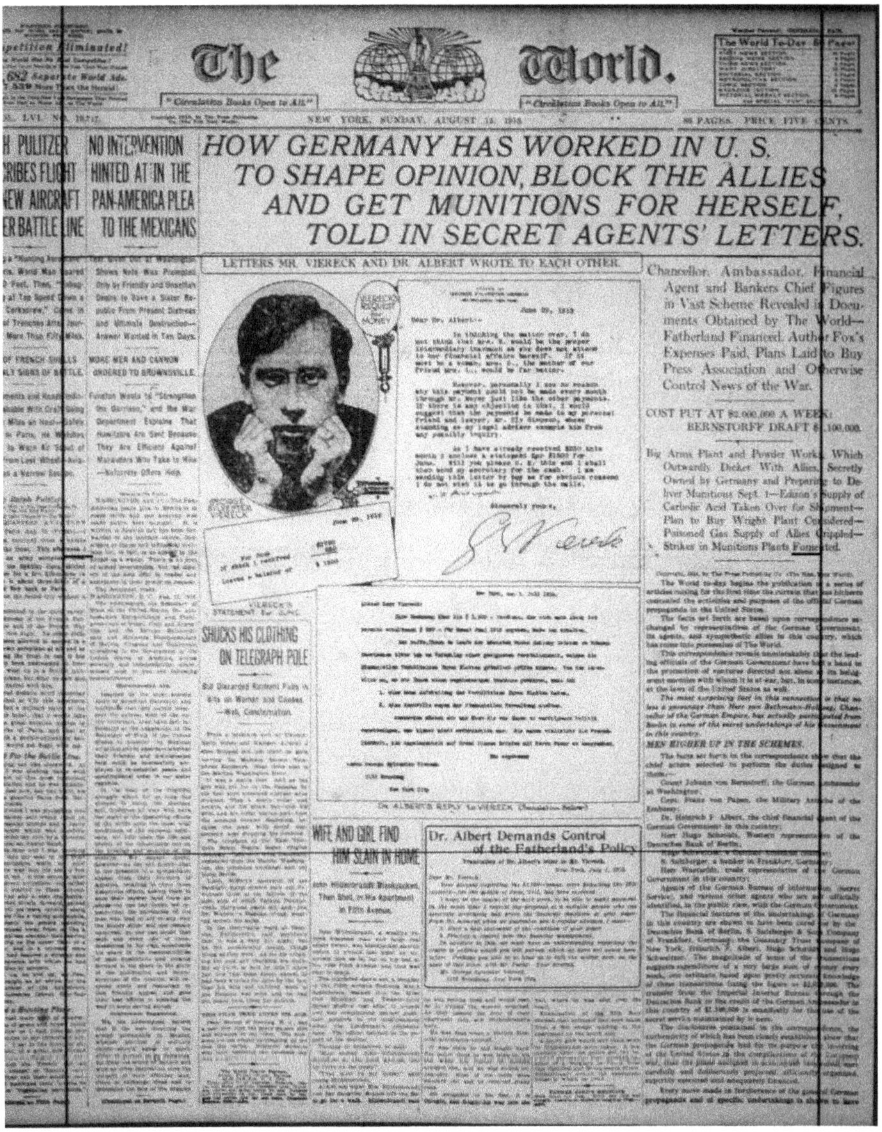

The World.

"Circulation Books Open to All."

NEW YORK, SUNDAY, AUGUST 15, 1915

NO INTERVENTION HINTED AT IN THE PAN-AMERICA PLEA TO THE MEXICANS

HOW GERMANY HAS WORKED IN U. S. TO SHAPE OPINION, BLOCK THE ALLIES AND GET MUNITIONS FOR HERSELF, TOLD IN SECRET AGENTS' LETTERS.

LETTERS MR. VIERECK AND DR. ALBERT WROTE TO EACH OTHER.

Chancellor, Ambassador, Financial Agent and Bankers Chief Figures in Vast Scheme Revealed in Documents Obtained by The World—Fatherland Financed; Author Fox's Expenses Paid, Plans Laid to Buy Press Association and Otherwise Control News of the War.

COST PUT AT $2,000,000 A WEEK; BERNSTORFF DRAFT $1,100,000.

Big Arms Plant and Powder Works, Which Outwardly Dicker With Allies, Secretly Owned by Germany and Preparing to Deliver Munitions Sept. 1—Edison's Supply of Carbolic Acid Taken Over for Shipment—Plan to Buy Wright Plant Considered—Poisoned Gas Supply of Allies Crippled—Strikes in Munitions Plants Fomented.

SHUCKS HIS CLOTHING ON TELEGRAPH POLE

WIFE AND GIRL FIND HIM SLAIN IN HOME

Dr. Albert Demands Control of the Fatherland's Policy

Figure 1-6: *'The great phenol plot' made the front page of the* New York World *on August 15, 1915.*

The story of aspirin's creation and rapid popularity provides several messages. The first is that the movement from antipyrine to aspirin reflects a microcosm of the history of the industry—moving from a plant-derived medicine to a synthetic product born of coal tar. The phenomenal success of aspirin also led Bayer and other companies to the realization that production of medicines could be highly profitable and spurred the continuing evolution of producing drugs from coal tar. Finally, the story of the Reverend Stone's discovery is a reminder that an incorrect theory can result in a good drug. The use of lithium in mania, for instance, originally came about while searching for a non-existent illness known as 'brain gout' (Chapter Five). Similarly, the use of bromides as sedatives was derived from the notion that excessive masturbation led to seizures, and that bromides were noted to decrease sexual interest[4]. Thus, Stone's belief in the now discredited 'doctrine of signatures' led him to emphasize the utility of the precursor of aspirin to the Western world.

'The arsenic that saves': Atoxyl and Salvarsan

Ehrlich's career in tissue staining had involved not only methylene blue and trypan red, but also an organic arsenic compound known as atoxyl. Later in 1905, when it was shown that Atoxyl was effective against the trypanosome parasites causing sleeping sickness (trypanosomiasis), Ehrlich chose to use it as a starting point for developing antimicrobials.

The history of Atoxyl began in 1859, when Antoine Béchamp, while working with aniline dyes, formulated it, describing it as 40 times safer than arsenic, which had been known for millennia as both drug and poison. It had some utility in stemming sleeping sickness in both humans and animals in Africa. To give a sense of the seriousness of sleeping sickness and the value of its treatment, sometime later in the 1920s, the Bayer company offered to give the British the structure of its drug, known as Bayer 205, in exchange for repatriation of German colonies ceded in World War I. Atoxyl, however, was far from benign. Robert Koch studied it in German East Africa and found that 2 percent of patients went blind from optic nerve damage.

In 1905, *Treponema pallidum*, the spirochete bacteria responsible for syphilis, had been discovered and was found to have a certain resemblance to the trypanosomes which caused sleeping sickness; one of the discoverers, Erich Hofmann, approached Ehrlich about developing chemical treatments. Syphilis, which may have been brought to Europe by the crews of explorers of the New World, spread rapidly, often on the coattails of wars in the fifteenth and sixteenth centuries*. Originally, as it proliferated through the continent, syphilis, often acutely lethal, was a much more virulent illness than it is today, possibly because it was new and there was little time for the population to develop resistance. By the

---

* There are two competing theories about this. The other view is that syphilis already existed in Europe, though unrecognized, prior to Columbus.

nineteenth century, some strains of the spirochete which produced less severe acute infections came to dominate, but syphilis remained a significant public health concern. As we will see in Chapter Three, its long-term consequences in the nervous system continued to lead to a significant portion of psychiatric hospitalizations.

Though the experience with Atoxyl was not promising, Ehrlich used it as a starting point in searching for medicines for syphilis. He and his colleague Alfred Bertheim clarified its structure in 1907, and Bertheim was tasked to synthesize variations on the molecule. Each subsequent compound was then tested for biological activity, using a model developed by the Japanese bacteriologist Hata Sahachiro in which rabbits were infected with spirochetes. In 1909, the 606th chemical was tested by the team and reported to have no value. Ehrlich, unconvinced, asked Hata to look into it further. It turned out to have some effect on trypanosomes, but to potently kill the spirochetes responsible for syphilis, prompting an irritated Ehrlich to revamp testing procedures. 'Compound 606,' arsphenamine, became available in 1910 as Salvarsan, 'the arsenic that saves,' a great improvement over inorganic mercury which had been widely used (see Chapter Four). Along with the improved Neosalvarsan, it was the dominant medical treatment for syphilis until it was replaced by penicillin in the 1940s.

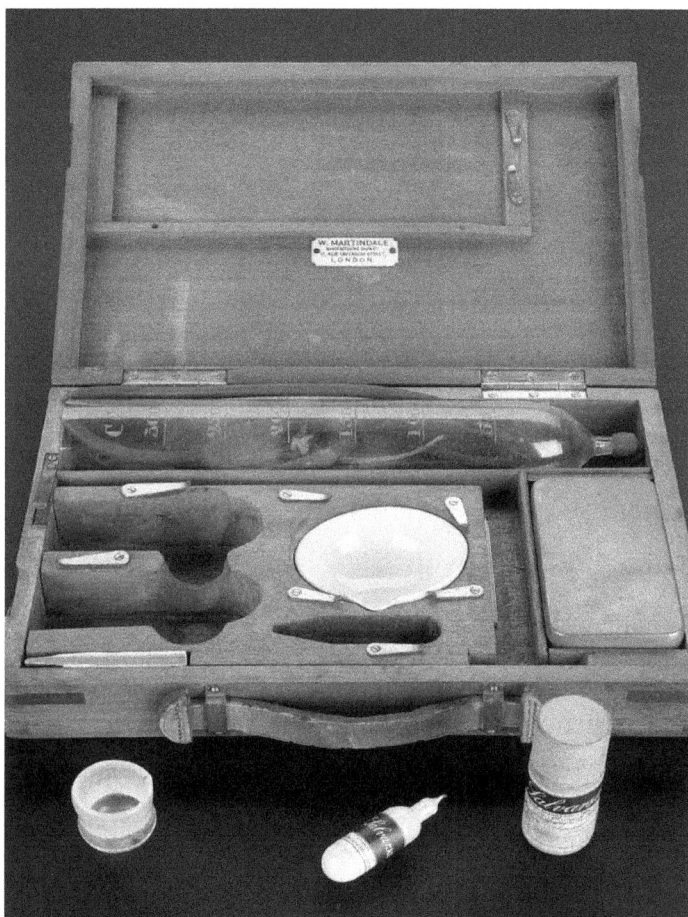

Figure 1-7: Salvarsan treatment kit, 1912. Although Salvarsan was a major step forward in treating syphilis compared to mercury compounds (Chapter Four), it was difficult to prepare and administer. Because it broke down in air, the ampules of yellow powder were prepared in carbon dioxide gas. It had to be carefully dissolved in large volumes of sterile water with minimum exposure to the atmosphere. Despite these limitations, after its introduction in 1910, its use rapidly spread and it shortly became the most commonly prescribed medicine worldwide at the time.

One unintended consequence of the success of Salvarsan was a series of accusations leveled against Ehrlich in what were known as the 'Salvarsan wars.' Just as James Young Simpson, discoverer of chloroform anesthesia for childbirth, had been accused of subverting biblical teachings, Ehrlich was said to have contributed to a loosening of morals. It was rumored that prostitutes were involuntarily given Salvarsan at Frankfurt Hospital. Ehrlich's Jewish heritage was invoked in complaints that he had profited excessively. The bacteriologist Paul Uhlenhuth, who had worked with arsenicals and later went on to be remembered for his many contributions but also his affiliation with the Nazis, claimed to have discovered Salvarsan first. Others emphasized the deaths that occurred while Salvarsan was being developed, implying that Ehrlich was ruthless. Though Ehrlich was exonerated in the sense that in 1914 a leading accuser was convicted of criminal libel, he continued to dwell on this as well as the outbreak of World War I. He became depressed and is said to have remained so until his death from a stroke the next year. It was a bittersweet end for a man who ultimately was honored with everything from a Nobel Prize to appearing on postage stamps and banknotes, and even having a crater on the moon named after him.

The story of Salvarsan was notable for several things. It was the first drug designed to deal with a specific microbe and was a major step forward in the treatment of the early and middle stages of syphilis. In a period which emphasized the immunologic approach to infectious diseases, in which Ehrlich had also been a pioneer, it cemented the role of drugs as well. Ehrlich coined the term 'chemotherapy' for the use of medicines to selectively kill bacteria or parasites while leaving the host unharmed, though it evolved to have a wider meaning today. Moreover, in developing a technique in which organic chemists would create variations on a lead molecule and then test the series of compounds for biologic activity, he had created a model which is used by pharmaceutical companies to this day. Examples of this approach include the discovery of the antipsychotic clozapine while searching for new antidepressants by screening modifications of the imipramine molecule; similarly, chlorpromazine was developed while screening chemical derivatives of methylene blue for use in malaria (Chapter Two).

As it turned out, Salvarsan had limitations as well, including a variety of side effects and difficulty in preparation and injection. It was also less effective for general paresis, one manifestation of the infiltration of syphilis into the nervous system which appears in the late stages of the infection, and which produced a significant portion of patients in psychiatric hospitals of the time. As we will see, a treatment for late-stage syphilis would come along later with the discovery of penicillin.

Prontosil red dye, sulfa drugs, and the first antidepressants

The story of sulfa drugs begins with Gerhard Domagk (1895-1964), born in the Brandenburg area to a schoolteacher and a mother from a farm family who later died of starvation in a refugee camp in 1945. He became a medical student, but after enrolling in the army with the outbreak of World War I, was wounded and transferred to the medical service. There he served in a cholera hospital in Russia, as well as various military hospitals where he became impressed with the deadliness of infected wounds. After the war and completing his medical degree, he taught at the University of Münster, and later moved to the IG Farben company, where he attempted to make antibacterial agents*. After a number of failures, he and his colleagues turned to an old technique for improving the attachment of dyes to wool by incorporating a sulfonamide group into azo dyes. One such compound which had previously been synthesized as a dye, out of the thousands tested over five years, was particularly effective in killing *Staphylococcus* and *Streptococcus* infections in mice. It was known as prontosil red and was patented in 1932 and given the trade name Prontosil. In the meantime, Domagk continued to have doubts whether this would translate into an effective antibacterial for humans. It was then that his daughter Hildegarde fell down some steps, in the process sticking her hand with a sewing needle and developed blood poisoning. When it seemed likely that her arm would have to be amputated, the

---

* I.G. Farben, the 'dye industry syndicate corporation,' was a conglomerate founded in 1925 and included the Bayer Company; after World War II it was dissolved, and the section which included Domagk became the newly re-established Bayer.

desperate father gave prontosil red to her, and within a week she was on the way to recovery. Convinced himself of its utility, he did not write about his daughter's experience but waited until 1935, when very positive clinical reports were published. He was met with a great deal of skepticism by the medical community, which, despite the success of Salvarsan, still tended to favor immunologic approaches and were skeptical of a chemical's utility in treating a generalized bacterial infection. The attitude toward Prontosil changed in 1936 when it successfully treated President Franklin D. Roosevelt's son of a very serious strep infection. In a way, its sudden fame was reminiscent of the popularity of aniline purple dye after Queen Victoria first wore her purple gown (see Prologue).

No sooner had Prontosil's use blossomed than it suddenly came to a standstill in 1937. Harold Watkins, a chemist at the S.E. Massengill Company in the U.S. created 'Elixir of Sulfanilamide' by dissolving it in diethylene glycol, a highly poisonous cousin of automobile antifreeze, and adding strawberry flavor and saccharin. Within a few months, over one hundred people died of kidney failure after drinking the Elixir, and the distraught Watkins committed suicide. In those years, there was no required testing of safety for new drugs, and the company was merely fined $26,000. One consequence of the tragedy was that in 1938 Congress passed the Food, Drug and Cosmetic act, which authorized the FDA to certify safety of new drugs, as well as cosmetics and medical devices. About a decade later, an analogous catastrophe occurred. In 1949, the widespread and unregulated consumption of lithium chloride as a salt substitute in the U.S. produced significant toxicity and even deaths, leading to a ban on lithium for this use (Chapter Five). By coincidence, this was the same year that Australian psychiatrist John Cade published his first reports of the effectiveness of lithium for bipolar disorder. The recent experience of lithium chloride as a salt substitute, however, led to the suspicion with which lithium for psychiatric purposes was treated and its slow acceptance into the medical community.

With time, sulfanilamide, the active component of Prontosil, regained favor. It was found that Prontosil was in fact what is called a pro-drug, that is, it is metabolized in the body to the antibacterial sulfanilamide, which has the antibacterial property. Eliminating the dye component had an additional benefit—one of the side effects of the original compound had been that it turned the skin red. Sulfanilamide in a powdered form was widely used to treat wounds in World War II. A number of other sulfanilamides were developed, as well as drugs with other purposes such as the diuretic furosemide. They remained the dominant antibacterials until the advent in the 1940s of penicillin, which was both more potent and was more benign in terms of side effects. Domagk's work did not stop with sulfonamides, however. Tuberculosis became widespread in Europe in the years after the end of World War II. Neither sulfanilamide nor penicillin were effective against tuberculosis, and Domagk set about the search for a new agent. While improving the effects of the sulfa derivative sulfathiazole, his work at the Bayer company laid down one of the trails to isoniazid, a tuberculosis drug used to this day, a derivative of which became the first modern antidepressant (Chapter Two).

In 1939, Domagk was offered the Nobel Prize, but Hitler had previously decreed that Germans could not accept it, after an experience a few years earlier in which Carl von Ossietzky, a critic of the regime, won the Nobel Peace Prize. He was briefly arrested by the Gestapo and forced to sign a document refusing the prize. After the war, he later was able to accept it in 1947.

CHAPTER TWO: THE TRANSFORMATION INTO MEDICINES IN PSYCHIATRY

Iproniazid: A tuberculosis drug and one of the first antidepressants

In the years after World War II, tuberculosis was rampant. The development of streptomycin was a major step forward, but its usefulness was ultimately limited both by its side effects, including deafness and vertigo, and by a growing resistance by the bacterium. In the race to find new treatments, the best-known story is the development of isoniazid from rocket fuel. During World War II, the Nazis devastated London neighborhoods with their V2 rocket, which in later years was fueled with a chemical known as hydrazine.

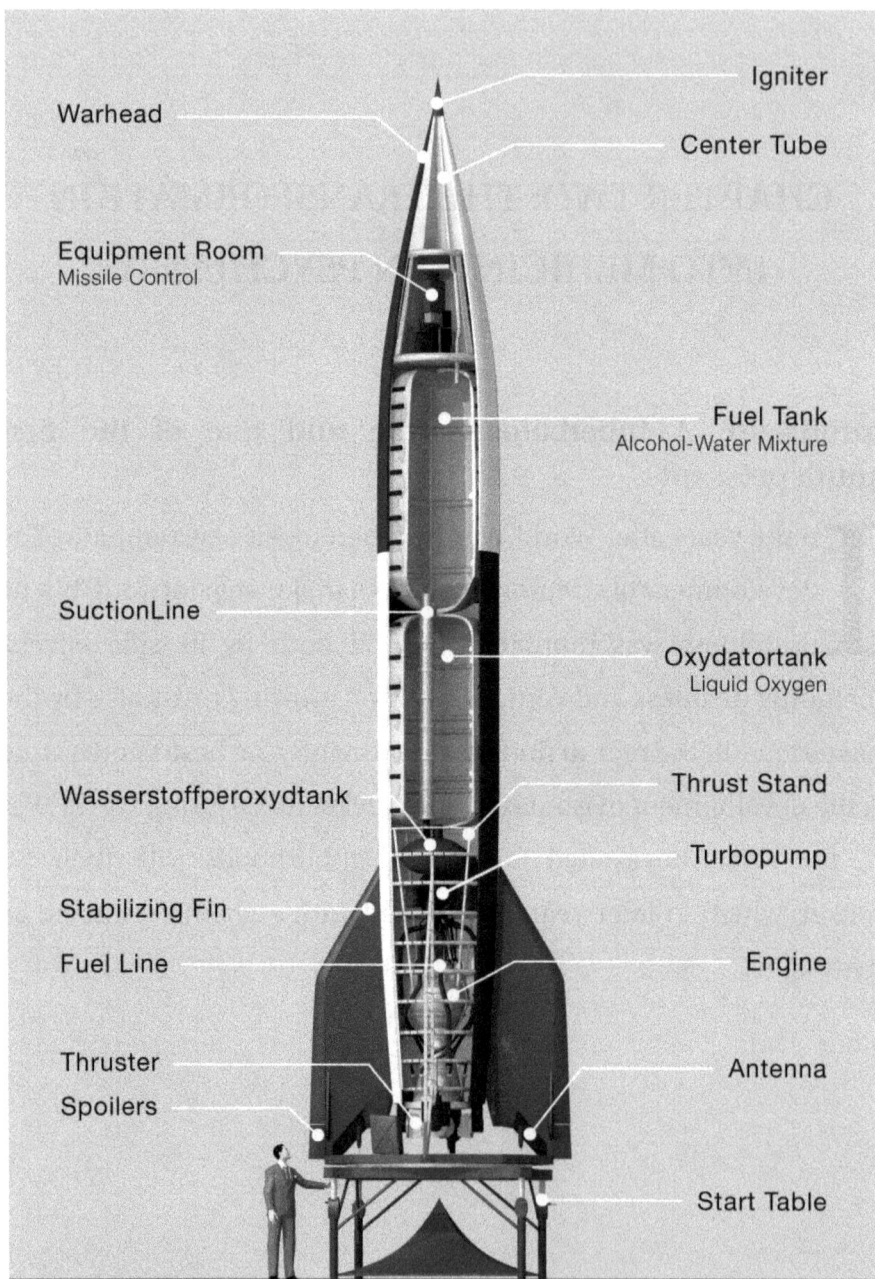

Figure 2-1: Diagram of the V2 rocket, the first guided ballistic missile, was originally fueled by alcohol and liquid oxygen, later replaced by hydrazine. The Nazis used it as a terror weapon against London and Antwerp, causing substantial

damage and loss of civilian life. It also became the first human-built device in space after being fired vertically in June 1944. Ironically, its hydrazine fuel later became one of the building blocks for both a new drug for tuberculosis and one of the first antidepressants.

At the end of the war, there was a large surplus of hydrazine, which was sold at bargain prices to industry. One of the buyers was the Hoffman LaRoche company, which believed it could be used as a building block for synthesizing medicines. This turned out to be the case, and in 1951 Roche scientists in Nutley, N.J. developed the anti-tuberculosis drug isoniazid and a related compound, iproniazid. It actually turned out that the story is more complex. In a remarkable coincidence, isoniazid was discovered around the same time in 1951 by the Bayer company in Germany, and Hoffman-LaRoche and Squibb in the U.S., using varying approaches[5]. Patent difficulties became moot when it was discovered that some Czech students had synthesized it in 1912, and all three companies developed it, though it was best known as Roche's product Rimifon in 1952. Although often recognized as a hydrazine derivative (its formal name is isotnicotinic acid hydrazide), there was more than one trail to its creation. A very important one was Gerhard Domagk's work trying to improve on the anti-tubercular action of the antibiotic sulfathiazole, in which he described in 1946 the potent activity of a group of compounds known as thiosemicarbazones. In doing so, he developed on of the important stepping stones to isoniazid (marketed by Bayer as Neoteben), for which he was cited in the Nobel award[6].

Iproniazid, the chemical cousin of isoniazid, was found to block the breakdown of the neurotransmitters norepinephrine and serotonin, and hence were known as monoamine oxidase inhibitors, or MAOIs. Early in the testing, it was noticed that tuberculosis patients receiving them, particularly iproniazid, had improvements in mood, energy, and appetite. Initially, it was thought that this might be due to improved nutrition, but ultimately this 'side effect' became much more evident, as in higher doses could lead to inappropriately euphoric mood or even psychoses. A trial at Staten Island's Sea View Hospital was widely publicized, with newspaper reports of very ill patients dancing in the halls. Though such accounts were perhaps exaggerated, psychiatrists including Nathan S. Kline (1916-1983) at Rockland State Hospital became interested and confirmed its utility in non-tuberculosis patients with depression. Iproniazid entered the market in 1958. Though later withdrawn due to liver toxicity, safer related compounds were developed. Thus, the MAO inhibitor iproniazid, derived from rocket fuel and sulfa antibiotic research, is remembered as one of the first modern antidepressants.

Chlorpromazine

How a failed antimalarial revolutionized psychiatry: Just as the discovery of iproniazid as an antidepressant hinged on a chance observation, so too did the discovery of the first modern antipsychotic result from an unexpected aspect of an aid to anesthesia. The story began in Bizerte, Tunisia, the northernmost city in Africa, and in the post-World War II years, the site of a major French naval facility. In the Bizerte Naval Hospital in nearby Sidi Abdallah was a young surgeon named Henri Laborit (1914-1995), born in colonial French Indochina, who had been decorated for his actions during the evacuation of Dunkirk. Laborit was interested in the problem of surgical shock, a complication in which a precipitous drop in blood pressure and circulation could often lead to a fatal outcome. He developed a theory that the body's response to surgical stress was a mixed blessing—although in some senses helpful, an excessive response might lead to shock.* Since the interaction with stress of anesthetics of the time, such as chloroform and ether, could also contribute to shock, he reasoned that drugs that might lower the dose of anesthetics would be beneficial as well. His focus was on the autonomic nervous system as well as histamine, which is released during surgery.

---

* The notion that a normally helpful physiologic process can be harmful in excess comes up in many other contexts. In psychiatry, anxiety in appropriate amounts is recognized as being useful—for instance, improving vigilance of potential hazards or as a spur to problem solving—but becomes deleterious when its magnitude is too great and inhibits functioning.

As it happens, a new class of drugs which block histamine's actions were becoming available around that time. In 1937, Daniel Bouvet[**] at Paris's Pasteur Institute had been interested in finding drugs which block neurotransmitters, which transmit signals between neurons. Three of them, acetylcholine, epinephrine, and histamine, had fairly similar structures. Since blockers for the first two had already been found, he reasoned that it might be possible to find one for histamine. He asked his student Anne-Marie Staub to give a variety of compounds to see if they interacted with histamine. The result was known as F929, which was found to save guinea pigs from the otherwise lethal effects of high doses of histamine. Though F929 was too toxic for human use, he had found the key to a new class of drugs. The clinically used antihistamine Antergan came out in 1942, followed by diphenhydramine (Benadryl and other brands) in 1945. The success of diphenhydramine led a group headed by chemist Paul Charpentier at the Rhône-Poulenc company to develop improved alternative antihistamines, in this case derivatives of methylene blue. Laborit tried one of them, promethazine, and found that it quieted presurgical patients and complemented the anesthetics.

In 1950, Laborit was transferred to the military hospital Val de Grâce in Paris, a former abbey going back to the seventeenth century, and

---

[**] In passing, he and his director Ernest Fourneau had also synthesized sulfanilamide, later developed into a clinical antimicrobial as we described in Chapter One.

continuing his interest in antihistamines, asked the Rhône-Poulenc company for any new related drugs. At the time, Charpentier's group was working on developing derivatives of methylene blue for the treatment of malaria and parasites. One of these, chlorpromazine, in a family of molecules known as phenothiazines, proved ineffective for this purpose, but Charpentier realized that it had significant antihistaminic properties, as well as quieting behavior in animals observed by his colleague Simone Courvoisier, and sent it on to Laborit.

Before long, Laborit and his colleagues found that as part of an 'anesthetic cocktail,' chlorpromazine was useful in surgery, decreasing the dose of anesthetics needed and lowering body temperature as well, in what he viewed as a kind of 'artificial hibernation.' He also made the unexpected observation that when given pre-surgically, it produced a state of indifference in patients, without necessarily putting them to sleep. He intuited that this might be useful for psychiatric purposes and contacted psychiatric colleagues at Val de Grâce. They gave chlorpromazine to Jacques Lh., a 24-year-old with mania. He rapidly became calm, though the effect decreased over a few hours. He was then given repeated doses of chlorpromazine as well as barbiturates, and within three weeks he was able to be discharged. The work with chlorpromazine was presented at a French medical meeting and published in 1952, but it was largely ignored by the psychiatric community, which emphasized shock treatment and psychotherapy for psychotic states.

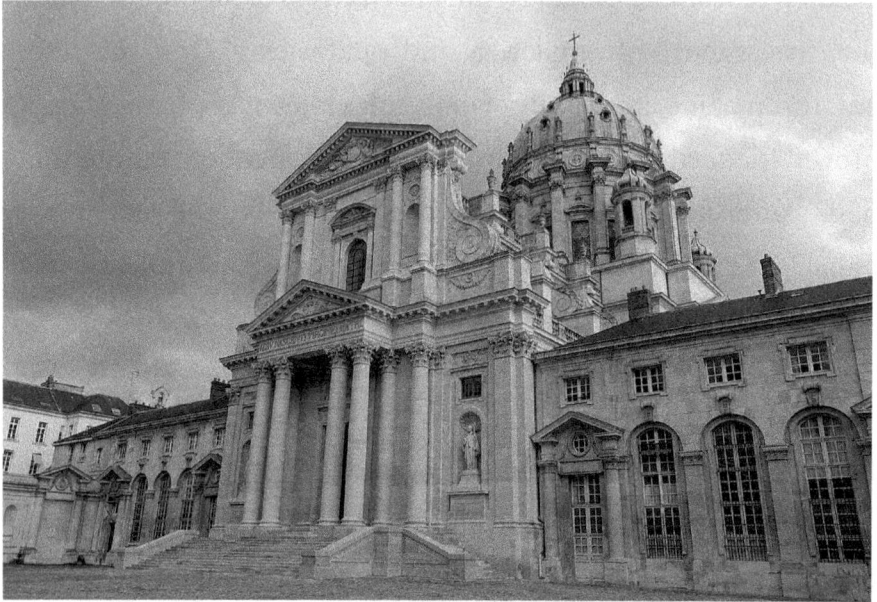

Figure 2-2: Val de Grâce, the military hospital in Paris at which Henri Laborit and colleagues first gave chlorpromazine to a psychiatric patient. It was originally built as a church in 1621 by Queen Anne of Austria, wife of Louis XIII, in gratitude for giving birth to Louis XIV after having been childless for 23 years. During the French Revolution, the nuns took care of sick or injured fighters, and a few years later it became a military hospital and is active to this day. Its dome is a well-recognized feature of the Paris skyline.

As it happened, one of Laborit's anesthetist colleagues was the brother-in-law of Pierre Deniker (1917-1998) at St. Anne, a large academic psychiatric facility in Paris. Deniker brought this to the attention of his director, Jean Delay (1907-1987), the son of a surgeon and a remarkable psychiatrist who also held degrees in literature and philosophy, and who in addition to his medical work had published novels and a biography of his friend, the writer André Gide. At that time, cooling with ice packs was one of the techniques used to quiet patients, and a drug that reduced agitation with inducing sleep and which lowered body temperature seemed promising. Deniker and Delay launched a series of studies of chlorpromazine in psychotic patients. They learned that it was effective in itself without the need of barbiturates, helping to not only calm agitated patients but reduce delusions and help bring order to disordered thinking processes. Moreover, they found that the cooling aspects of the drug were not essential to its function. Before long, their studies were echoed by other European groups, and in 1952, chlorpromazine was marketed in France with the brand name Largactil ('large in action'). Within a few years, it was well-recognized internationally. Patients who previously would have needed to be hospitalized were able to be treated in clinics; many who had been hospitalized were now able to be discharged. There were problems as well—often communities were not prepared to accept the large numbers of previously hospitalized patients—but the discovery of chlorpromazine led to optimism that new drugs could be found to treat the most severe psychiatric disorders.

Laborit himself went on to discover some of these new medicines. In 1958, he built a laboratory at Boucicaut Hospital in Paris and went on to develop the sedative clomethiazole, the MAO inhibitor minaprine, and wrote about the relation of biology to social problems such as dominance and aggression. His laboratory was primarily supported by income from his drug patents. Like John Cade, who re-discovered lithium treatment for mania (Chapter Four), most of his work was done outside traditional universities. His strong belief in challenging traditional viewpoints earned him the antipathy of the medical establishment—indeed, Jean Delay went to Stockholm to argue against him receiving the Nobel Prize—but was the foundation of his extraordinary career.

How chlorpromazine led to the tricyclic antidepressants and the antipsychotic clozapine: Chlorpromazine led to interest in developing chemically similar compounds which might have antipsychotic effects. As we mentioned in Chapter One, methylene blue, and chlorpromazine from which it was derived, are considered phenothiazines, the chemical core being comprised of three ring-like, or tricyclic, structures. The Geigy company produced a number of variations and sent them for testing in psychotic patients. One of them developed in 1950, known as G22150, reached Roland Kuhn (1912-2005), a psychiatrist working at a lakeside hospital in Münsterlingen, Switzerland. It became too expensive to use, and when Kuhn asked for alternatives, he was sent one called G22355. In the earlier study, he had noted that the mood had improved in some patients with psychoses with depressive features, and that others had developed euphoria. Perhaps for this reason, or the coincidence that his hospital was unusual in having an outpatient facility, or even from a sense of thoroughness, he gave it to depressed patients. In 1956, he reported on three patients whose mood improved when on the medicine, worsened when it was stopped and got better when it was resumed. Following a 1957 paper on a much bigger study, the drug imipramine was marketed in Europe and later in the U.S. in 1959. It was the first of what came to be known as the tricyclic antidepressants.

The success of imipramine, in turn, led other companies to study variations on the molecule. One of them, the Swiss company Wander AG, came across a group known as 'neuroleptic tricyclics,' which had chlorpromazine-like properties in animal behavioral testing. One of them seemed to be less sedative and, interestingly, also made them less sensitive to pain. These qualities led to developing it further for human use, and ultimately it became an antipsychotic named clozapine. The surprising thing, though, is that it later turned out that the animal pain studies had been in error, the result of electrodes which had short-circuited. Though one of the reasons it had been developed was spurious, clozapine became a very useful drug. One of its side effects related to suppressing white blood cells slowed its acceptance, but after approval by the FDA with a set of safety monitoring precautions in 1989, it became recognized as a drug which often helped in persons who had not improved with chlorpromazine or other 'typical' antipsychotics. In a sense, then, the circle was complete: the antipsychotic chlorpromazine led to the antidepressant imipramine, which in turn led to the antipsychotic clozapine.

Benzodiazepines: unsuccessful azo dyes grew into blockbuster tranquilizers

Leo Sternbach (1908-2005) was the son of a pharmacist, born in what is now Croatia. After a number of moves due to the hard times after World War I, the family settled in Krakow, Poland. There he enrolled in the University of Krakow, which was closed to Jews, but which made an exception because his father had become a prominent pharmacist before the closing. He earned his PhD in organic chemistry and taught there until his position was transferred to a non-Jewish Polish chemist in 1936. After some interim work, he moved to Switzerland in 1940, where he went to work for the Hoffmann-La Roche company in Basel. In 1941, when Germany invaded Greece and Yugoslavia and the situation felt more insecure in Switzerland, the company moved its headquarters to the U.S. Using travel documents provided by Roche, Sternbach and his wife escaped through France and Portugal, settling near the company's laboratories in Nutley, New Jersey. He was known as a good chemist, but his habit of criticizing his bosses led him to be passed from one group to another. Fortunately, early on he found the first commercially successful method for synthesizing biotin (vitamin B7), which was included in multivitamin products; in this sense, he was like Alexander Fleming, who had already one major discovery (the antibacterial enzyme lysozyme) before the later discovery which made him famous (Chapter Three). The discovery was also valuable for Sternbach politically; it secured his place while he lobbied to have more freedom in his work.

At the time, the success of meprobamate in 1953 (see Chapter Three) led Sternbach's superiors at the Hoffman LaRoche laboratories to ask him to work on developing new tranquilizers. Since several companies were working with small alterations on the meprobamate molecule, his task was to find an entirely new approach. In choosing his starting materials, he recalled that during his training in Krakow, he had studied azo dyes and derivatives called 4,5-benzo-[hept-1,2,6-oxdiazines]. At the time, they had not been found to have good prospects as commercial dyes, and the work had been discontinued, but in retrospect he realized that they might be good building blocks in his new work. He proceeded to synthesize about 40 variations on these molecules, but on animal testing most did not appear to have the profile of tranquilizers. His boss began to feel that this would not be a fruitful project and reassigned him to work on antibiotics. That would have been the end of the story, but later, in 1957, one of his assistants was cleaning out old unused bottles and found one which apparently was the 40th, untested compound from his previous work. He asked Sternbach if it was okay to toss it out. Instead, Sternbach, who had been told to do other work, asked his colleagues to do animal testing on this one last sample. When the skeptical pharmacologists did so, it turned out to have sedative and muscle relaxant effects, and to differ from chlorpromazine, as it did not significantly alter autonomic nervous system function. Testing in larger animals showed that it decreased aggression. Studies from the San Diego Zoo described combative monkeys who became docile, and a bellicose lynx who became playful as a pussycat. A well-known collage released by the company shows a 40-pound lynx with a ferocious expression in one frame, and in the next docilely sniffing a flower. The first study in humans involved high doses and made patients dizzy, with slurred speech. Roche interested Irvin Cohen, a private psychiatrist in Galveston, Texas, to use lower doses in outpatients, and he and two others reported success in decreasing anxiety, improving sleep, and giving a sense of well-being. As time went on, thousands of patients were studied in formal clinical trials.

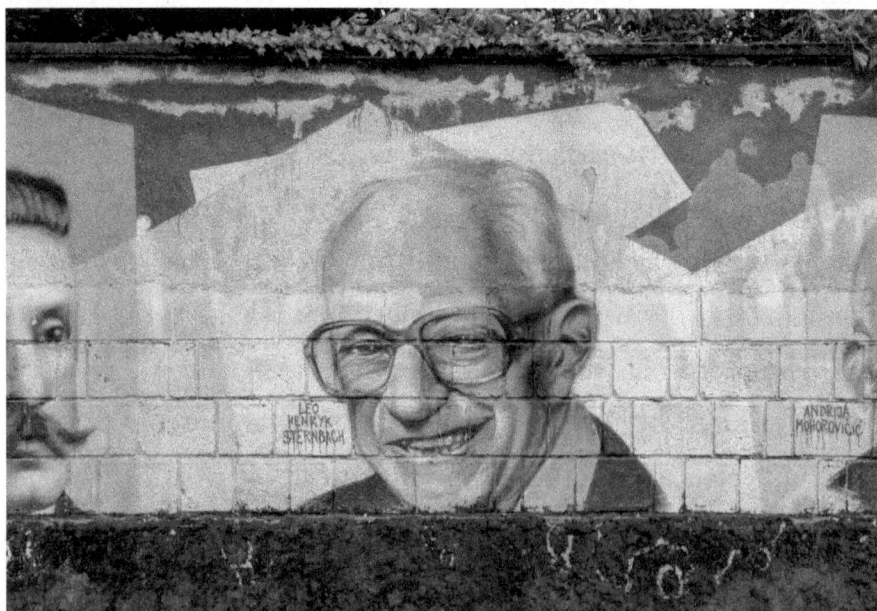

Figure 2- 3: Leo Sternbach's fame spread back to his hometown in Opatija, Croatia, where this graffiti picture of him appeared in 2019.

Sternbach re-evaluated the chemistry of the compound, chlordiazepoxide, and determined that it was in a family known as benzodiazepines, which as the name suggests, were formed from the combination of a benzene ring with a diazepine nucleus. It was marketed in 1960 as Librium (as in 'Equilibrium') and was followed a few years later by Valium (in which the 'Val' came from the Latin *valere*, to be strong). He continued to develop new variations, and like John Cade with lithium (Chapter Four), he tested some on himself. On one notable occasion, a new prospective drug left him bed-ridden for two days, evoking in his wife 'a little scare.' His work produced seven more benzodiazepines, and ultimately about a dozen were marketed by various companies for use as tranquilizers, sleeping agents, muscle relaxants, anticonvulsants, and sedatives during procedures such as colonoscopy and mechanical ventilation. Their success was phenomenal, and by 1977 they were the most widely prescribed drugs in the world.

Much of the initial popularity of benzodiazepines came from the perception that they were much safer than the then-dominant barbiturates. With time, though, their many limitations also became apparent. They were classified as Drug Enforcement Administration Schedule IV controlled substances, and reports came out of impaired driving, as well as confusional states in the elderly. In 2016, the FDA issued a 'black box' warning of their potentially lethal effects when combined with opiates. For these reasons, treatment shifted to the newer selective serotonin reuptake inhibitors (SSRIs) for anxiety and the 'Z drugs' such as zolpidem for sleep. But the story of the beginnings of the benzodiazepines, with their subsequent rise and later decline, began with a persistent chemist finding a new use for azo dyes.

As for Sternbach, he continued a productive career, developing other kinds of drugs as well, including ones to treat high blood pressure, and to minimize bleeding during brain surgery, ultimately holding 241 patents. Even though his discoveries led to 40 percent of the company's sales at one point, he never became wealthy, earning one dollar per discovery, the fee paid to him for turning over the patent rights to his employers. But this never seemed to be his goal, which was freedom to pursue studies in medicinal chemistry. Even after his retirement in 1973, he worked as a consultant, coming to the office almost every day until two years before his death at the age of 97.

CHAPTER THREE: INFECTIOUS DISEASES AND PSYCHIATRY

In the Prologue, we touched on how William Henry Perkin stumbled upon aniline purple dye while trying to synthesize quinine, and Chapter One described how Paul Ehrlich recognized the anti-malarial properties of methylene blue. Actually, malaria is so interwoven into the story that it's worthwhile to look at its history and relevance to psychiatric illness, and how medicines for it were developed from other dyes. In Chapter One, we also described Ehrlich's discovery of Salvarsan, the first effective treatment for syphilis. Here we will follow this up with a description of the relevance of neurosyphilis to psychiatry, the remarkable consequences of its treatment with penicillin, and how an investigation of penicillin preservatives accidentally led to the first modern tranquilizer.

'Bad air'—the story of Malaria

Malaria is an infectious disease which causes intermittent fever and chills, headache, muscle pains, fatigue, and yellowing of the skin, which can progress to stupor, coma, and lethality. Currently about

228 million people around the world suffer from it, resulting in over 400,000 deaths annually. It is due to several species of microscopic *Plasmodium* parasites, which are transmitted to humans by infected *Anopheles* mosquitos.

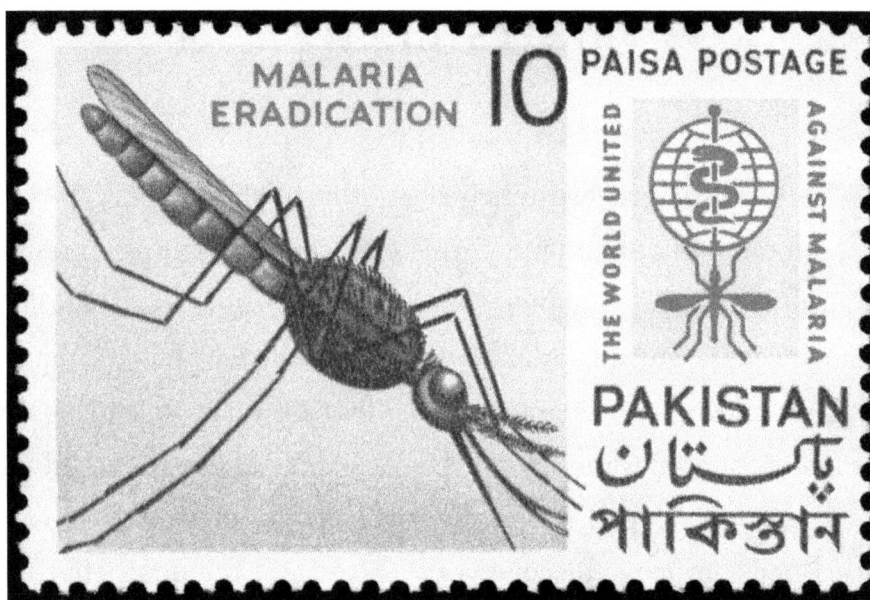

Figure 3-1: The Anopheles *mosquito, as pictured on a Pakistani 10 paisa stamp. After being bitten, the first signs of illness often appear about two weeks, and initially can be hard to identify as malaria. Treatment in the first 24 hours is important to prevent progression of the illness. Children are the most vulnerable and account for about two-thirds of deaths. Unless adequately treated, it may reappear months later, though usually not as severe. If not re-exposed, a person with partial immunity may become vulnerable again as the years go on.*

Plasmodium parasites have been found in mosquitos embedded in amber 30 million years ago. There is evidence that malaria began to significantly affect human health in the Neolithic period, or New

Stone Age, about 10,000-12,000 years ago, during a time of transition from lives of hunting and gathering to the development of agriculture. Over the centuries, humans developed genetic mutations which provided some resistance to malaria, and which remain to this day in the form of illnesses such as sickle cell disease and thalassemia. Malaria greatly hindered the building of the Egyptian pyramids. It is mentioned in Homer's epic *The Iliad* from the eighth century BC, and later in the works of the classical Greek playwrights Aristophanes and Sophocles. Some authors believe that it contributed to the diminution of the ancient Greek city-states, and later weakened the Roman Empire, where there was a general belief that it arose from the foul air of nearby swamps. This led sometime later to the word malaria, from the Medieval Latin *mal aria* ('bad air'). Malaria continued to affect Italy during the Renaissance and is said to have felled a number of the princely Medici family. In England, it was called marsh fever and overlapped with the vaguely described condition of 'ague.' It was a prominent enough concern that it appeared in *Gulliver's Travels* and *Robinson Crusoe in the 18th century,* and later *Treasure Island* and *Great Expectations* in the 19th century. Malaria was a problem for the British Army in the south during the American Revolution and hindered the process of empire building worldwide. It is not surprising, then, that finding a treatment was much on the mind of scientists at the Royal College of Chemistry in the 1850s (see the story of William Henry Perkin in Chapter One). It was not until the 19th and early 20th century that the association of malaria with mosquito-borne parasites was understood, and the modern era of widespread use of insecticides and swamp draining was initiated. Still, to this day, 40 percent of people globally inhabit malaria-prone areas.

Psychiatric complications of malaria: During World War I, a great deal of attention came to be focused on psychiatric consequences of malaria, which had been known for some time but came to the forefront in the Balkans Theatre. There were vivid accounts of amnesia, confusion, and manic-like behavior[7], as well as coma accompanied by other neurological signs in what came to be known as 'cerebral malaria.' Milder forms were associated with insomnia, irritability, and mood disorders; in other cases, patients were hospitalized with confusional psychoses, and only later with the development of fever was malaria recognized. At one point, these kinds of complications of malaria were the most common kind of psychiatric morbidity among the troops in Macedonia. During World War II, when malaria was a serious problem for troops in Africa and the Pacific (Chapter One), psychotic states were reported, as well as complaints of residual memory difficulty after treatment. Many years after the Vietnam conflict, soldiers who had had malaria were found to have a variety of neurocognitive deficits as well as mood disorders and alterations in personality. In more recent years, a large population study in Kenya found an association of 'common mental disorders,' though not psychoses or PTSD, with positive blood tests for malaria parasites.[8] An understanding of the relation of such disturbances with malaria is made more difficult by the frequent psychiatric side effects of synthetic antimalarial medications such as chloroquine.[9,10]

'Jesuit's bark,' the Countess of Chinchón, and quinine

The discovery of coffee's cousin: It seems likely that malaria was brought to the New World by Europeans, and possibly by their African slaves. It was also in the age of imperial expansion into the southern hemisphere that the first widespread treatment for malaria, the source of what later became the drug quinine, appeared. There are several stories of how this came about. Peruvian Amerindians ground up bark from the 'quina-quina trees' in the misty slopes of the Andes for reducing fevers, as well as for controlling the chills from being cold, long before the arrival of Europeans introduced malaria. In one legend, reminiscent of the story of the Reverend Stone discovering the benefits of willow bark for his ague (Chapter One), a feverish native drank from a pool of water, even though it had a bitter taste coming from the surrounding quina-quina trees, and found relief. Seventeenth century missionaries in Peru saw Amerindians using quina-quina bark in the areas where the tree flourished, often at altitudes above 1500 meters[11], too high for the *Anopheles* mosquito to prosper and hence less likely to have endemic malaria[12,13]. Though this indigenous use was likely for other types of fevers, or for chills from a cold environment, the missionaries tried and found it beneficial for malaria in the lowlands. 'Jesuit's bark,' as it came to be known, was brought back to Europe by the missionary Bernabé de Cobo

(1582-1657), and by the 1700s it was established to be effective relatively selectively for malaria and came into wide use.

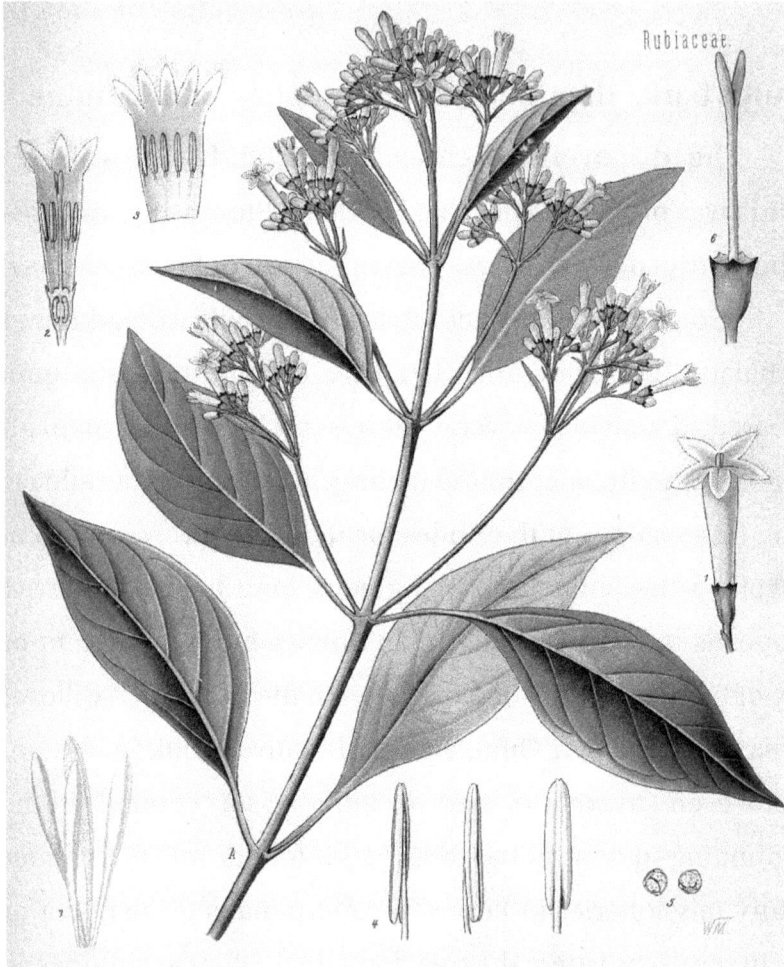

Figure 3-2: Cinchona officinalis, *as depicted in this 1887 print, was likely the tree whose bark was called quina-quina, from the Inca name 'holy bark,' and became the source of quinine. It was employed since antiquity by the indigenous Quechua people in the Peruvian Andes to relax muscles and combat shivering in the cold environment, often taken by dissolving it in sweetened water to help cover its bitter flavor, much as the British did in their far-flung colonies in the eighteenth century, in the form of tonic water.*

The story is often told (and also questioned by some later historians) that the wife of the Spanish Viceroy of Peru, the Fourth Count of Chinchón, became ill with malaria in the early 1600s and was successfully treated with cinchona bark. The grateful patient is said to have then brought the bark back to Europe, and in 1742 the famous Swedish botanist Carl Linnaeus (1707-1778) named the genus of the trees *Cinchona*, part of the Rubiaceae family which also includes coffee plants. There is also some evidence that it was actually another tree, Peruvian Balsam (*Myroxylon peruiferum*), that was prized for a bark which relieved fever and was widely imported to Europe. In this version, fraudulent importers debased it by adding *Cinchona* bark which appears similar and was apparently easier to obtain. Ultimately, what began as an additive was recognized as the active ingredient for malaria.

Regardless of its origins, quinine was discovered as the active ingredient and was named by the French scientists Pierre Joseph Pelletier and Joseph Bienaime Caventou in 1820. The importation of bark became a very active business, and in order to maintain their monopoly, Peru, Ecuador, and Bolivia forbade taking seeds or plants out of the county, while in the meantime native trees were being harvested without replanting. In the 1850s and 1860s, the Dutch managed to get plants which they sent to Java, while a British expedition did the same and carried them to India and Sri Lanka. In 1864, an Englishman, Charles Ledger, and his attendant Manuel gathered a quantity of seeds of a particularly valuable type of *Cinchona*. They were caught by the Bolivians, and Manuel received a thrashing from which he never recovered. Ledger in the meantime sent the seeds to his brother in London. They were shown to the British, who were not interested; the Dutch quickly bought them and forwarded them on to Dutch Indonesia, where *Cinchona ledgeriana*, as the plant came to be called, turned out to be much more productive of quinine than previous kinds. Ultimately, the Dutch effectively controlled most of the world's supply of quinine, much as they had done with rubber.

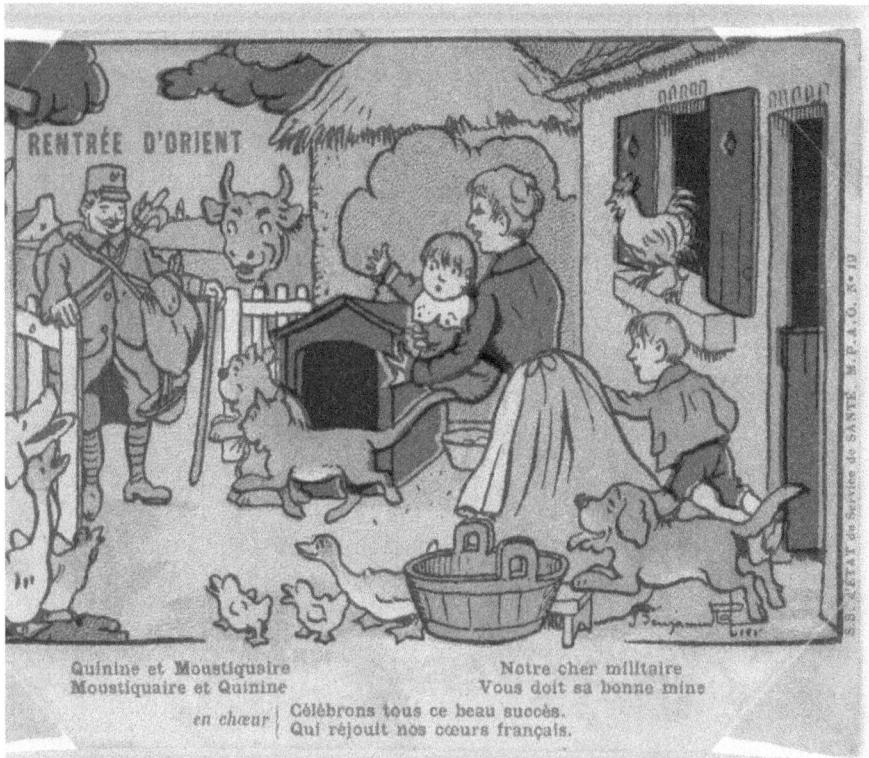

RENTRÉE D'ORIENT

Quinine et Moustiquaire
Moustiquaire et Quinine

en chœur

Notre cher militaire
Vous doit sa bonne mine

Célèbrons tous ce beau succès.
Qui réjouit nos cœurs français.

Figure 3-3: In this illustration by Benjamin Rabler (1864-1939), a French soldier is returning to his family from the East. The text indicates that quinine and mosquito netting are responsible for the French army's looking well and celebrates their success. Rabler was also a comic book and commercial artist. His most famous creation was La vache qui rit, 'The laughing cow,' whose smiling face first adorned processed cheese in 1921 and remains popular today.

The quinine missions of World War II: After Pearl Harbor, America was essentially cut off from its source of quinine, and there was a scramble to find replacements. Seeds from the Philippines were grown in Costa Rico. In 1942, the U.S. Board of Economic Warfare organized a group to explore local sources of *Cinchona* bark in South America. Led by University of Michigan botany professor William C. Steere, the party consisted of foresters, botanists, and a lawyer (the latter seemingly unusual in the annals of the profession). They began their expedition in the higher altitude Colombian rainforests, identifying *Cinchona* trees, and testing for their yield by means of a process in which ground bark was heated in a test tube; if pink smoke appeared, it was evidence of a good quinine yield. An additional mission was sent by the American Quinine Company to Ecuador in 1943. It was led by an anthropologist, who was joined by Steere. Both groups sent harvested bark which was carried by hand or on mules, and ultimately it found its way by rivers or bush planes to base laboratories or was shipped directly to the U.S. The missions produced significant amounts of quinine for American troops and along the way discovered new species of *Cinchona*.

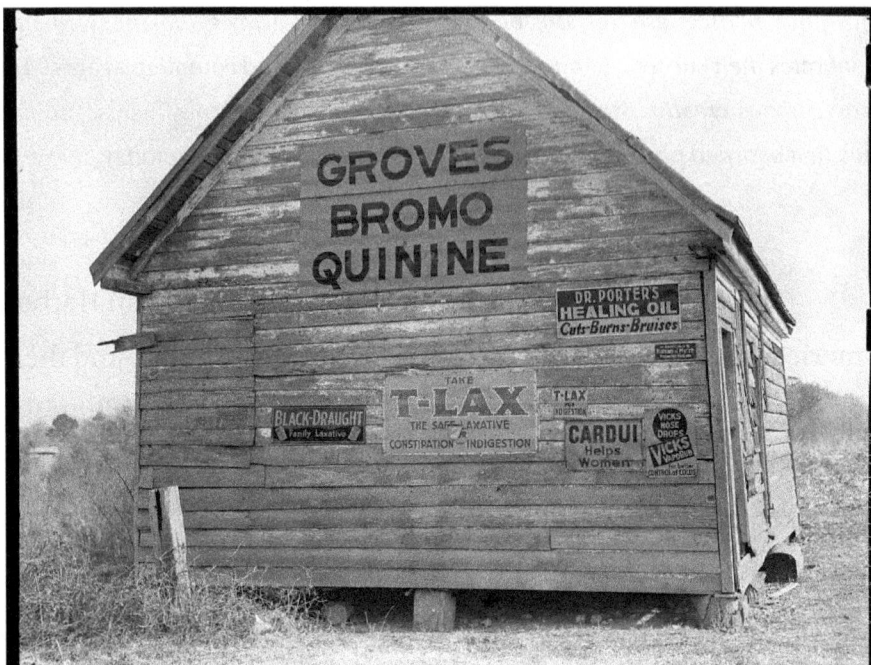

Figure 3-4: Advertisement for quinine, 1938. Malaria has been endemic in the South from the earliest days of colonization. It hampered the British Army during the revolution, and the Union Army during the Civil War, and continued to be a problem through the 1940s. The predecessor of the Center for Disease Control (CDC), the Office of Malaria Control in War Areas, was established in 1942 and was located in Atlanta rather than Washington DC, in recognition of the impact of malaria in the South. By 1951, the occurrence of endogenous malaria in the U.S. became less common, though still not fully eradicated, and is the subject of active surveillance.

Dye derivatives to the rescue: synthetic drugs for malaria

Although the quinine missions yielded a valuable supply of *Cinchona* bark, there was still not enough. As we described in Chapter One, the military also used methylene blue, which though not as effective as quinine, was of some help. They also turned to synthetic drugs. In 1931, the yellow acridine dye derivative quinacrine (also known as mepacrine or the brand name Atabrine) had been developed from methylene blue, as a synthetic replacement for quinine, and was distributed to troops in World War II. Interestingly, American spies infiltrating Japanese-occupied China used quinacrine to change their Caucasian skin coloration to look more Asian. Quinacrine's use was limited by side effects including ringing in the ears, skin itching, difficulty with balance, liver toxicity, depression, and psychotic states (presumably not very desirable in the practice of spy-craft).

Quinacrine was later replaced by chloroquine, created in 1934 essentially by removing one of the three benzene-like rings in the structure. It was initially discarded by Bayer as having too many side effects, in what came to be known as the 'Resochin error' (referring to a brand name). It was reconsidered in the U.S. a decade later, becoming widely used around 1947, and continues to be prescribed. Though yellow skin coloration is uncommon, its side effects include damage to the retina, nerve-type hearing loss, and seizures, as well as a variety of other medical and psychiatric consequences[14]. It can also be a cause of methemoglobinemia, due to excessive amounts of an abnormal kind of hemoglobin, resulting in blue coloration of the skin in Caucasians (Chapter Five). Chloroquine was followed in 1955 in the U.S. by hydroxychloroquine, a variant which also carries risk of damage to the retina and heart muscle and psychiatric disturbance. The artemisinins were derived in the 1970s from *Artemisia annua*, the sweet wormwood plant traditionally used as a Chinese herbal medicine. Interestingly, in the last decade, methylene blue has been re-evaluated for having a role in malaria treatment, possibly by augmenting the effects of quinine and chloroquine[15].

As for quinine itself, 124 years after it was identified, and 88 years after Perkin's first attempts to produce it (Chapter One), American chemists Robert Burns Woodward and W.E. Doering were able to fully synthesize it in 1944. Even though later improvements were made, it was never turned into an economic industrial process and continues to be obtained from *Cinchona* bark. It is still available as a minor drug for malaria, and in the past has been used off-label for nighttime leg cramps though later the FDA issued a 'black-box' warning against this practice. One legacy it leaves behind is its use in tonic water, originally developed because British colonials in the tropics found quinine's taste so bitter that they dissolved it in soda and sweetened it with sugar. It found its way into mixed drinks such as gin and tonic and is still available, though with reduced amounts of quinine. To this day, tonic dispensers in bars are often labeled with a 'Q' in memory of its origins.

Malaria treatment for neurosyphilis

Although the advent of Salvarsan in 1910 had been a major step forward in the treatment of syphilis, one of its limitations was its lack of effectiveness for general paresis, one of the consequences of syphilis invading the nervous system, often decades after infection. Because of this long lag time, it wasn't clear until 1913 that it was associated with the spirochetes of syphilis. Symptoms included personality changes, emotional instability, memory deficits, hallucinations, and dementia, culminating in progressive fatigue and debilitation, usually with a fatal outcome within five years. Because of the many psychiatric manifestations, general paresis accounted for 10-45 percent of patients in psychiatric hospitals in the first half of the twentieth century. Probable victims ranged from all parts of society, from the philosopher Friedrich Nietzsche to Al Capone (both of whom may also have suffered from the toxicity of mercury treatments). Interestingly, in 1917, malaria also became involved in the treatment of neurosyphilis.

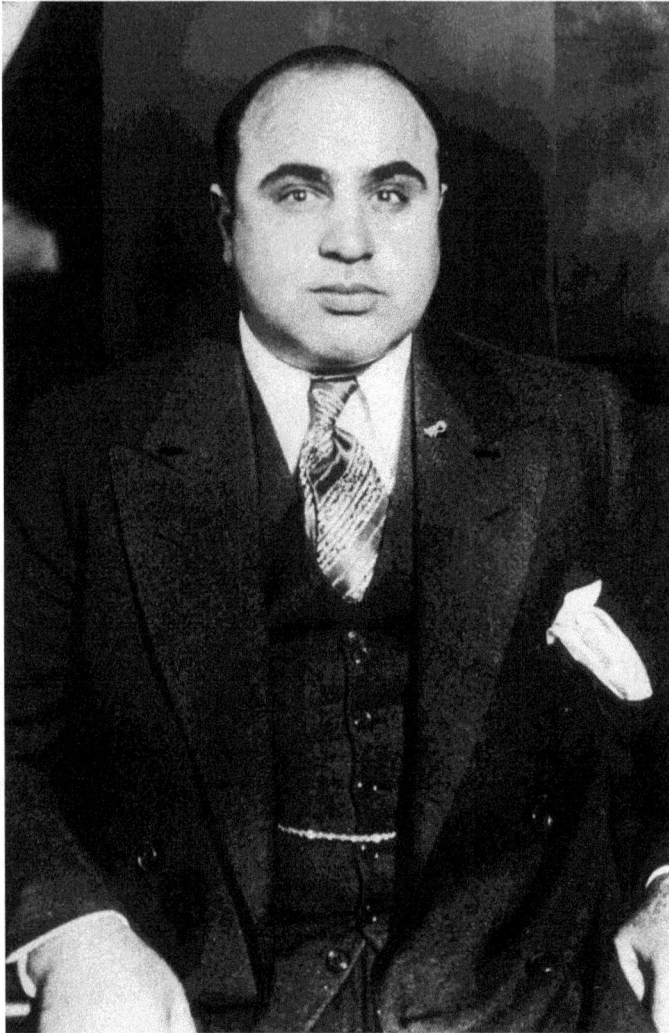

Figure 3-5: *Al Capone (shown here in 1930) eluded the clutches of the FBI, but not those of the Internal Revenue Service or the Treponema pallidum. In 1939, he was released from prison in view of his decline due to general paresis, and in 1942 at a very late stage in the disease was one of the first Americans to receive penicillin. The degree of injury to his brain was already so great that though it slowed down his deterioration, he never recovered, and died in 1947.*

The recognition of possible beneficial effects of malarial fever on psychiatric and neurological disorders goes back to antiquity. Reduction in epileptic seizures was observed by Hippocrates, the Greek father of medicine, and improvement in melancholy was described by Galen, the notable physician and philosopher in the Roman Empire. These and much later reports in the nineteenth century captured the interest of a young Austrian psychiatrist, Julius Wagner-Jauregg (1857-1940), who found that some general paresis patients greatly improved after febrile illnesses. Around 1887, he began purposely inducing fever with tuberculin, a mixture of proteins derived from the tuberculosis bacillus (still used today in the PPD skin test for TB), with unclear results. In 1917, he reported significant improvement in neurosyphilis patients who had been purposely infected with malaria while being monitored carefully in a hospital setting. The treatment became widespread (indeed, he won the Nobel Prize for it in 1927), often in combination with neurosyphilis medicines such as Salvarsan and penicillin) and was concluded by treating the malaria with quinine. Efforts to use this approach for other disorders such as schizophrenia had mixed results, but at the time this was considered a major advance in dealing with general paresis and remained so until it was eclipsed by penicillin in the late 1940s. Despite his Nobel Prize, Wagner-Jauregg has little recognition today compared to his fellow Austrian psychiatrist Sigmund Freud, in part perhaps for unwholesome associations during old age in 1930s Germany.

The accidental discovery of penicillin

In contrast to Wagner-Jauregg, Alexander Fleming (1881-1955), the discoverer of penicillin, is well known to this day. Born the son of a farmer in Ayrshire, Scotland, he came to London at age 13 and began work as a shipping clerk. There he might have remained, but as it happened, when he was 20 his uncle John Fleming left him an inheritance. Convinced by his older brother, a physician, to study medicine, he attended St. Mary's Hospital Medical School and later became caught up in World War I. He served on the Western Front, and later worked in an army hospital which had taken over the casino in Boulogne. There he studied what came to be known as evolving wounds, describing the changes in their appearance and secretions over time. His work is still recognized and earned him a place in medical history had he never discovered penicillin. He also took the controversial view that the antiseptics of the time, such as carbolic acid, iodine, or hydrogen peroxide, were harmful rather than helpful when applied inside wounds, as they could injure tissues and kill superficial bacteria but inadvertently allowed for growth of more toxic microbes deeper inside. The notion was resisted by battlefront doctors of the time, who had limited alternative resources available, but came to be generally accepted over the years. And it set the stage for Fleming to continue to pursue alternative approaches to fight bacteria.

After the war, Fleming returned to St. Mary's, where he became a professor of bacteriology. In 1922, while working with petri dishes containing bacterial colonies, he made a chance discovery. In one account he had a cold and placed some of his nasal mucous in a petri dish and apparently forgot about it. Two weeks later, he noticed that the place where his secretions were in the dish was surrounded by a clear area, indicating that bacterial growth on the plate was inhibited. He concluded that something in the mucous had weak antibacterial properties, and he went on to discover a substance called lysozyme, present in other fluids such as saliva, tears, and milk, which helps protect against infections. It turned out to be an enzyme which helps break down a constituent of bacterial cell walls, and its presence in saliva may be one of the reasons humans and animals instinctively lick wounds. However, its physical properties, and a narrow range of bacteria with which it was effective, limited its potential as a systemically given drug.

In September 1928, he had a similar experience which changed the world. Returning from a two-week vacation in Scotland, he noticed that one of the petri plates containing *Staphylococcus aureus* bacteria, which was supposed to have been placed in an incubator, had accidentally been left on a lab bench and become contaminated with airborne spores of a white fluffy mold. In the areas surrounding the mold, the bacteria samples turned transparent and were dying. Thinking back to his 1922 experience, he thought that something in the mold was toxic to the bacteria. Though this idea was not new—the ancient Egyptians had placed moldy bread on wounds, and the observation that bacteria could not survive near *Penicillium* had been made in 1870 by the English physiologist John Burdon-Sanderson—it was the first modern formulation of the thought, and the first to ultimately lead to extracting from its yellow juice the substance responsible. He called it penicillin, after the *Penicillium notatum* mold it came from. In one sense he was well prepared for the discovery—it was the culmination of his longstanding interest in natural substances with antibacterial properties, as well as his desire to treat wound infections. In some ways, though, these endeavors may have also limited his understanding of penicillin's potential. In 1929, Fleming published a paper about it, with only a minor reference to 'its possible use in the treatment of bacterial infections,' and there it remained, primarily as a tool for bacteriologists classifying penicillin-sensitive and penicillin-insensitive organisms. Though he thought penicillin might have some use in local application to wounds (continuing his interest in antisepsis from the war) or contaminated surfaces, he moved on to other things, in much the same way as John Cade after his studies of lithium treatment (Chapter Four). Surprisingly, for some time he believed that the discovery of lysozyme had been his most important finding[16]. (One is reminded of Arthur Conan Doyle, who believed that he should be remembered for his non-Sherlock Holmes novels, and that the stories of the famous detective were more of a diversion.)

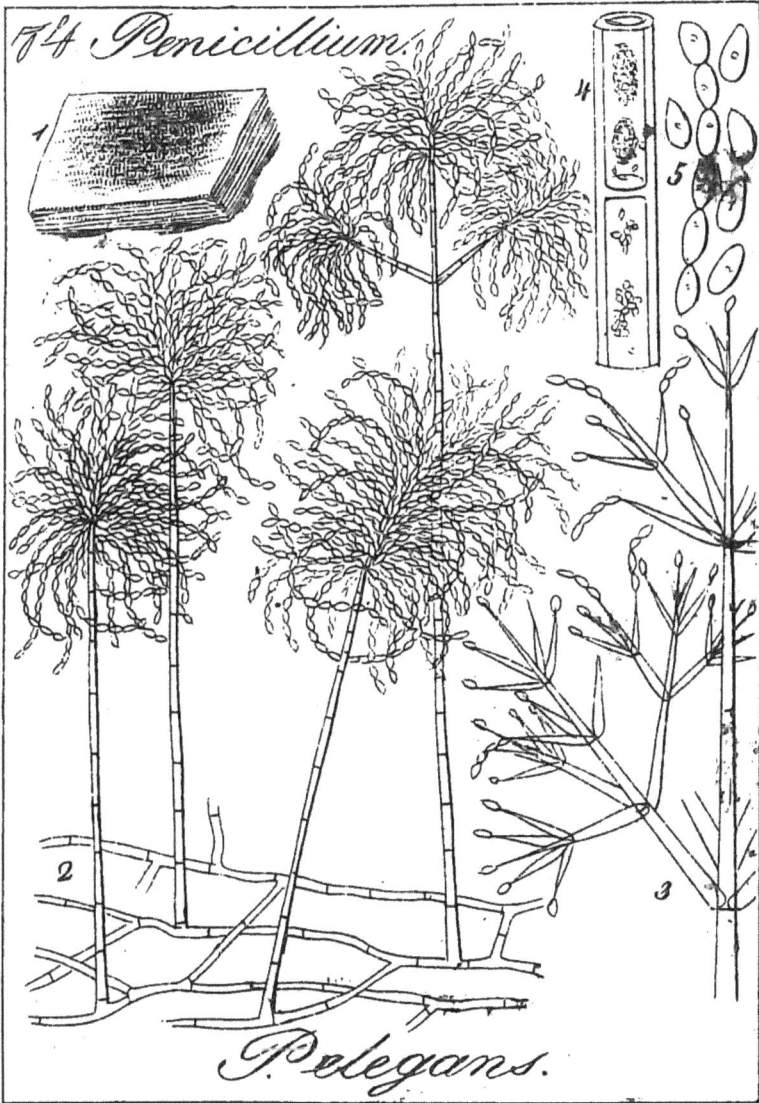

Figure 3-6: Penicillium *as drawn from a microscope in 1838. This particular one is* Penicillium elegans, *which grows in soil or on decaying wood, and is not harmful. The Penicillium genus contains about 300 species, including some used in making Brie, Camembert, and Roquefort cheeses.* Penicillium notatum *is the species Alexander Fleming first found contaminating his petri dish, which led to*

the discovery of penicillin. The drawing is from the work of A.C.J. Corda (1809-1849), a Czech doctor and scholar of fungi.

A decade later, in 1938, Howard Florey, an Australian and the director of the pathology department at Oxford, was pursuing his interest in how molds and bacteria affect each other, when he came across Fleming's article and saw its potential as a systemic antibiotic. In a way, the world had changed since Fleming saw limited used for penicillin. When he wrote his first article in 1929, there was general skepticism that medicines might be developed to treat infections throughout the body. With the advent of the sulfanilamides in 1936 (Chapter One), this now seemed possible. Setting up a team with biochemists Ernst Chain and Norman Heatley, Florey began the process of more carefully identifying the substance in mold juice, confirming that it prevented deaths from infection in mice, and dealing with the formidable task of producing it in quantity. By 1940, they felt ready to give it to a patient. Over dinner, Florey had heard about Albert Alexander, a 48-year-old policeman who had scratched his face while tending his roses, and developed abscesses in his eyes, scalp, and face, with spreading infection to his lungs. Though treatment with sulfa had been unsuccessful, he started to get better over a five-day course of penicillin. Then the supply ran out, and ultimately Alexander relapsed and passed away.

Spurred on by the initial improvement of the patient, the team struggled to produce penicillin in quantity but had limited resources in wartime England. Florey flew to the U.S. and convinced the U.S. Department of Agriculture to help in the effort. Aided by the chance discovery by Mary Hunt, an assistant in a USDA laboratory, of a more productive mold growing on a cantaloupe she had bought in the market, production began to increase. Penicillin made in the U.S. was first successfully given to a woman with a bacterial blood infection in March of 1942, exhausting half the existing supply. In June 1942, there was only sufficient penicillin in America for 10 patients. By June of 1944, over two million doses were available for use in treating wounds at the D-Day landings in Normandy.

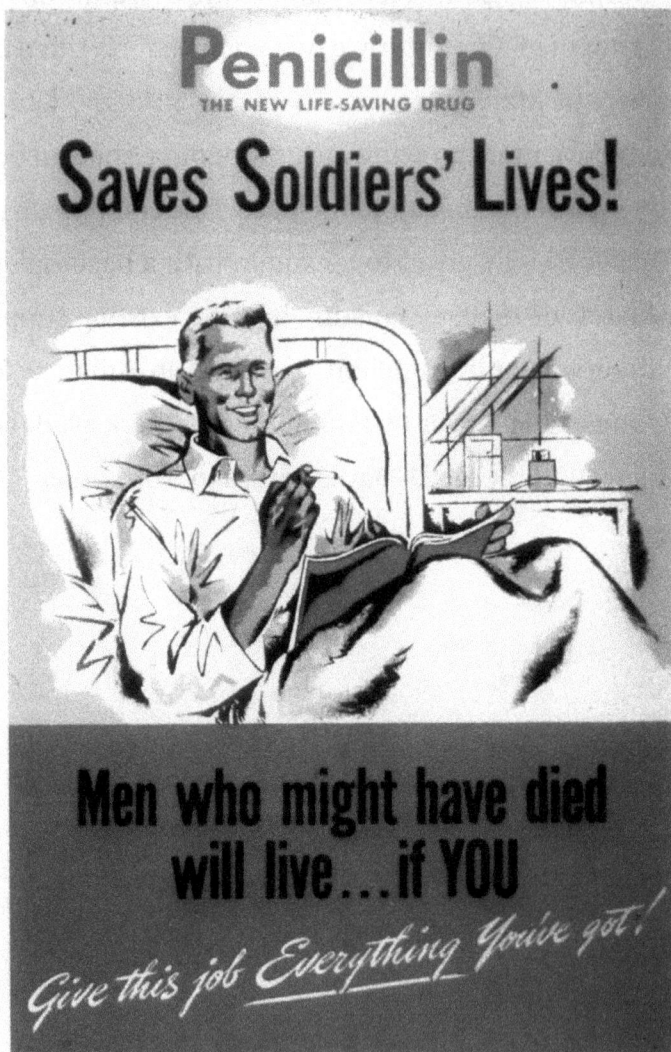

Figure 3-7: An American penicillin poster during World War II.

The impact of penicillin on psychiatry: After the war, as penicillin became available for widespread use, it was given to hospitalized neurosyphilis patients, with remarkably successful results. It quickly replaced malarial fever therapy and eliminated the need to hospitalize what before had been a significant portion of the inpatient population. This also resulted in several changes in psychiatrists' thinking. For one thing, the success of a drug in treating psychoses brought the hope that there might be more in the future. Secondly, it turned their focus from what were then known as 'organic' psychoses to 'functional' psychoses such as schizophrenia. Both the interest in new medicines and the change in focus culminated in the clinical discovery of chlorpromazine in the early 1950s (Chapter One). Both drugs, each in their own way, affected the number and types of patients requiring long-term inpatient care.

A second result of penicillin on psychiatry came from one of its limitations—as originally formulated, it was unstable, and could itself be broken down by enzymes secreted by bacteria which might get into the solution. For this reason, the development of preservatives went hand in hand with its expanded use. As we will see in the next section, it was while trying to find a useful preservative that Frank Berger stumbled upon what ultimately became the first modern tranquilizer. Afterwards we will talk about yet another consequence of penicillin, its place in shifting the way in which antibiotics would be developed in the future.

Meprobamate—an unexpected consequence of penicillin: Frank Berger (1913-2008) was born in West Bohemia (now the Czech Republic) and received a medical degree from the University of Prague in 1937. His interest was in laboratory work in basic pharmacology but was interrupted when, like Leo Sternbach (Chapter Two), he fled the Nazi occupation of Eastern Europe, settling first in England and then the U.S. While in England, he served as a physician in refugee camps, and he then went to the Yorkshire laboratory of the British Drug Houses, a group of dye and pharmaceutical firms going back to 1714 which had come together in 1908. His assignment was to develop a preservative for penicillin. While doing so, he noticed that one of them altered the behavior of rats and mice—they became much quieter, though still easily aroused. It occurred to him that this might be a useful drug for humans. He had long been interested in anxiety and had wondered about the physiology of how it could come and go at different times. In looking into his drug further, he found that indeed a very similar compound, mephenesin, was already on the market as a muscle relaxant during surgery and reportedly had anti-anxiety effects. As Berger saw it, mephenesin also had a number of limitations: it was very short acting, and its effects on muscle relaxation were relatively greater than its effects on anxiety.

Coming to the U.S. in 1947, he eventually settled at Wallace Laboratories in New Jersey, where he and a chemist, Bernard Ludwig, started with mephenesin and, using organic synthesizing techniques, came up with meprobamate in 1950. He had a difficult time selling the idea to his bosses, though; their poll of doctors had indicated little interest in a medicine for anxiety. Unlike William Henry Perkin, who went off and set up his own laboratory (see Prologue), Berger instead made a film of the effects of meprobamate on monkeys and showed it at a medical meeting. It got a lot of attention, leading his bosses to relent, and Miltown (named after the borough in New Jersey) was marketed in 1955, with immediate success. Reports came in of reduced anxiety in outpatients, as well as improvements in hospitalized patients and persons abusing alcohol. It captured the public's imagination and was frequently talked and joked about by television personalities, much the same as Viagra was for a later generation. By 1957, one-third of all prescriptions written in the U.S. were for meprobamate, and it became the first 'blockbuster' drug in psychiatry. It also led to a change in the way psychiatry was practiced. While chlorpromazine (Chapter Two) was originally oriented to helping hospitalized patients, meprobamate was a drug very suitable for office practice.

In time, it became clear that meprobamate was a mixed blessing. It was found to interfere with driving ability, to be liable to abuse, toxic in overdose, and to have a barbiturate-like withdrawal syndrome. In 1970, it became a Schedule IV controlled substance. With the advent of the benzodiazepines in the 1960s (Chapter One), interest in meprobamate languished and, though still available, it is rarely prescribed. But its history, born from an effort to find an agent to preserve penicillin and developed from organic compounds through the use of synthetic chemistry, was once again an example of the interaction of microbiology and psychiatry.

Penicillin and the transition in how antimicrobials are discovered: Penicillin was also emblematic of a change in the way drugs to fight infections were developed. So far, we have primarily described how medicines such as Salvarsan and sulfanilamide were created by synthetic organic chemistry. In the 1940s, there began to be an emphasis on discovering derivatives from soil bacteria. Streptomycin was one of the first. Like meprobamate, it is a New Jersey story, the work of Selman Waksman of Rutgers University, who had been looking at derivatives from *Streptomyces* bacteria which were toxic to other microbes. After the active substance streptomycin was isolated by his graduate student Albert Schatz, the new antimicrobial was successful in animal studies, and then in treating the first patient, 'Patricia T.' for tuberculosis in 1944-1945. A large study of infections in an Army hospital after the war had a less promising beginning—the first patient died, the second had blindness attributed to the drug—but the third was completely cured. As it happened, he was Robert J. Dole, who went on to become the Senate Majority Leader, running for president in 1996.

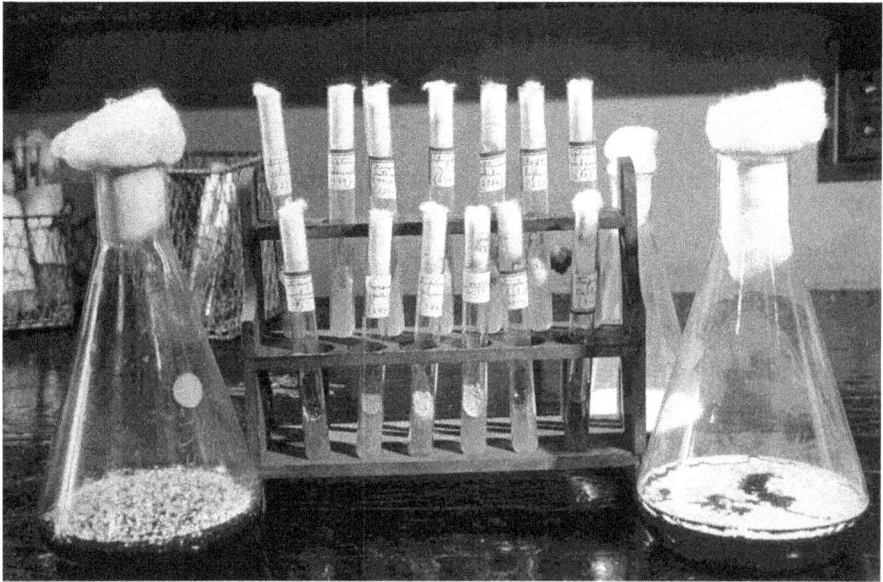

Figure 3-8: Cultures of Streptomyces griseus *bacteria in the Waksman Laboratory at the Agricultural Experimental Station of Rutgers University. Streptomycin, derived from the bacteria, interferes with protein synthesis in microbes, leading to their death, and has been successfully used for treating a number of diseases. Because it was discovered in New Jersey, legislators initiated a bill in 2017 to make* Streptomyces griseus *the official New Jersey state bacteria.*

Ultimately, streptomycin went on to become actively used for tuberculosis, usually given in combination with isoniazid (Chapter Two) or other drugs, as well as a variety of disorders including tularemia, plague, and endocarditis. As we described earlier, it was shortly followed by penicillin, a product of a mold, as well as the discoveries of chloramphenicol in 1947 and tetracycline in 1948 from soil bacteria. They all fell into the category of 'antibiotics,' a term Selman Waksman had coined in 1941 to refer to substances produced by microbes which in turn are toxic to other microbes. The techniques pioneered by Paul Ehrlich in making Salvarsan were greatly improved. While Ehrlich's team screened hundreds of substances before success with the 606th one, now millions of compounds can be screened. The enzymatic reactions inside bacteria are also often inherently more efficient than many multi-step organic syntheses, producing much higher yields.

As a result of these changes, the century-long interacting evolution of making dye-derived organic molecules into medicines for both microbiology and psychiatry declined in the 1940s and 1950s, as the two fields began to take their own paths forward. In one sense, this brings to an end the original story we set out to tell. The next chapters elaborate on two final points: One shows that it's never quite so simple—inorganic molecules were also found to be the source of useful drugs in both microbiology and psychiatry. The second describes how methylene blue and other dyes continue to be found to have new uses in medicines to this day.

CHAPTER FOUR: IT WASN'T SO SIMPLE—THE ROLE OF INORGANIC COMPOUNDS

Although we have focused on the importance of organic compounds in the evolution of modern drugs, it's worthwhile to mention that some inorganic compounds have been developed over the years and have played important roles. We will look at two of many examples: mercury compounds in general medicine, and lithium in psychiatry. Others which could have been selected include bromides, which were among the early sedatives, and bismuth, an early treatment for syphilis, now still used for traveler's diarrhea.

Mercury

The history of mercury as a medicine—and awareness of its toxicity in higher quantities—goes back to antiquity in Egypt and China. Qin Shi Huang, a Chinese emperor of the third century BC, whose physicians fed him large amounts as the key to immortality, reportedly went mad and suffered an early death at age 49. Even to the end he was a believer, and he was buried in a bejeweled tomb with mercury pools, which to this day cannot be opened because of concerns of toxic contamination. Cinnabar (mercury sulfide), the ore from which most pure mercury is extracted, appears in various hues of red, and when ground up became the original source of the pigment vermillion until synthetic ways were developed. It was used as a coloring agent over the centuries in cultures as diverse as the Mayans, who decorated burial chambers with it, the Song dynasty Chinese, who infused it into their lacquerware, and Western culture, which incorporated it into Medieval illustrated manuscripts. It is still found to this day in Chinese traditional medicine for sedation and other purposes. Cinnabar was widely used by the classical Greeks and throughout the Western world through medieval times for a variety of conditions including melancholy, venereal diseases, parasites, trachoma, and constipation. Mercury turned the stools black, and it was thought that this resulted from removing an excess of bile, one of the four 'humors' whose appropriate balance was believed to be important to health. On the contrary, excessive doses can cause difficulties with vision and hearing, kidney complications, peeling skin, itching or burning feelings of the limbs due to nerve damage, and memory and mood disturbances.

Both topical and oral forms of mercury were a mainstay in the treatment of syphilis, which had become widespread in Europe by the end of the 15th century. Calomel, a mercury chloride preparation, was in widespread use from the 16th until the early 20th century, as a cathartic, as well as for syphilis, typhoid fever, mumps, and a variety of other conditions. The administration for syphilis was immortalized in a famous saying: 'A night with Venus, and a lifetime with mercury.' Benjamin Rush, a physician and politician who had signed the Declaration of Independence, advocated calomel for mental disorders, as well as for yellow fever when it became widespread in Philadelphia in the late eighteenth century. Abraham Lincoln in his pre-presidential years took mercury pills known as 'Blue mass' for headaches. In those days, the usual amount of mercury contained in Blue mass was roughly one hundred times the current EPA guidelines. Some authors have suspected that one aspect of Lincoln's severe depressions and fits of anger, as well as physical symptoms such as difficulty walking and tremors, may have been toxic consequences. It is said that Lincoln may have seen the connection and decreased or stopped its use after the election. During the Civil War, William A. Hammond, the Union army Surgeon General, advocated limiting the administration of calomel to the troops, as he believed that adding dehydration from its cathartic properties, as well as the risk of mercury toxicity, was not of benefit to already-ill soldiers. He became very unpopular with army physicians, who often had few other resources for treatment available, and ultimately was fired. In retrospect, this may have had a silver lining: he moved to New York, became one of the first American physicians to specialize in mental disorders, and wrote reports of using lithium bromide as a treatment for manic episodes.

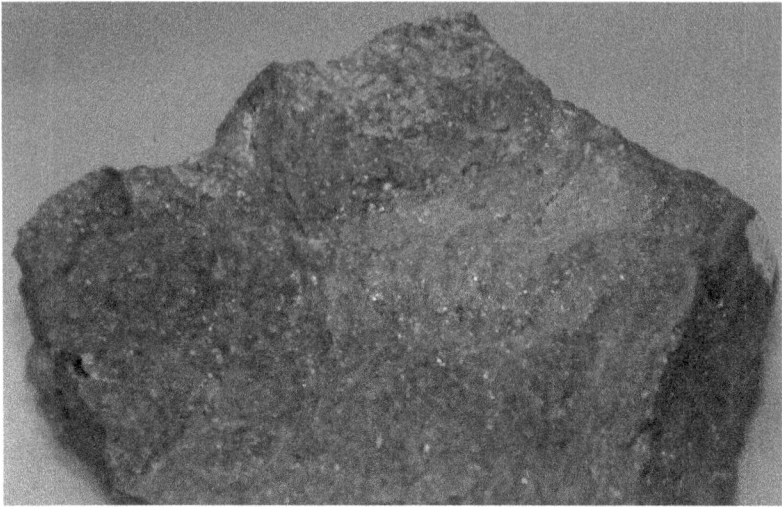

Figure 4-1: *Cinnabar, the main source of metallic mercury, is a mineral found in areas of volcanic activity and mineral hot springs. It has been used as a coloring agent as far back as the 10th century BC and found its way as vermillion dye into cosmetics, jewelry, and lacquerware. Often it was associated with blood or victory, and it was featured in ancient Roman processions. Cinnabar is significantly toxic and no longer used for decorative purposes, replaced by synthetic vermillion dye.*

Mercury had a place in the popular imagination as well. In Jules Verne's novel *20,000 Leagues Under the Sea*, the submarine *Nautilus* was powered by batteries containing mercury in combination with sodium from sea water. In the late nineteenth and first half of the twentieth centuries, mercury found wider and wider uses. The colorful bottles of liquids typical of apothecary's windows usually contained calomel, mercury oxide, cinnabar, or related compounds. Mercury products were widely used during both world wars, both as components of cartridge primers and blasting caps, but also as wound antiseptics. Organic preparations of mercury were developed in the 1920s and widely given as diuretics until the advent of the thiazide diuretics in the 1950s. Mercurochrome, an organic preparation, was a common over-the-counter antiseptic and is still used in some parts of the world though no longer in the U.S. Thiomersal, a mercury-based preservative, was widely used in vaccines, but it became a subject of controversy because of allegations of an association with autism; though most rigorous studies questioned any such relationship, it was banned or very greatly reduced in virtually all vaccines given to children. In summary, mercury, though plagued from the beginning with concerns about toxicity, was one of the inorganic substances with a long history in medicine.

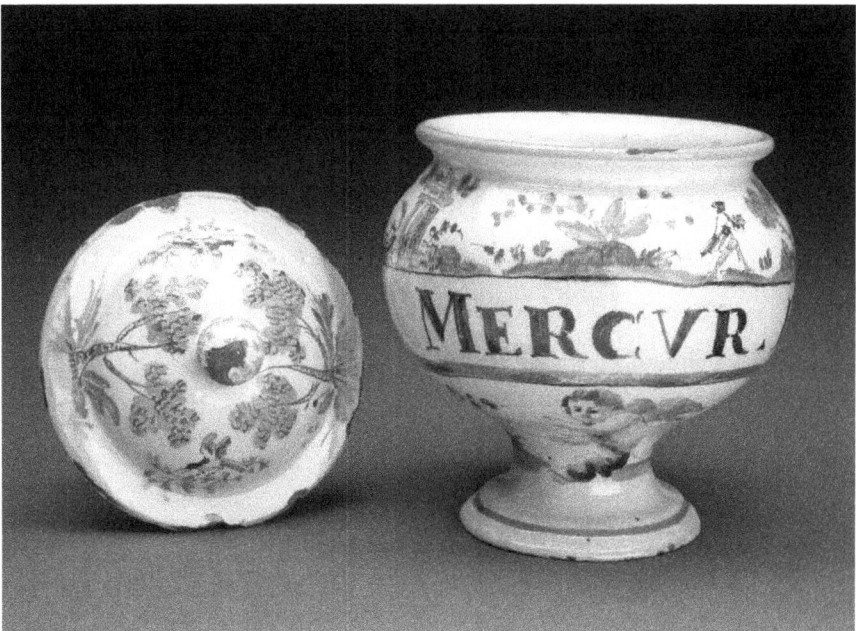

Figure 4-2: Decorative jar for mercury pills, Italy 1731-1770. The pills were probably from a formula invented by Augustin Belloste (1654-1730), who kept the ingredients secret, and whose family became very wealthy. Though fairly toxic, they were used for syphilis, kidney stones, and gout, and were still in circulation until the early 1900s.

Lithium

The histories of lithium and gout are closely intertwined. Gout is one of the oldest known diseases, described by the ancient Egyptians and the Greek physician Hippocrates. Though rare in most animals, it may have even afflicted 'Sue,' the well-known *Tyrannosaurus rex* dinosaur whose skeleton is on display in the Chicago's Field Museum. In humans, it is a painful inflammatory arthritis, characterized by nodules on the ankle, toe and heels. The name derives from the Latin word *gutta* (for 'drop') because it was believed that an excess of one of the four humors led it to drop into the joints, producing the nodules. In 1679, Antoni van Leeuwenhoek, the legendary Dutch microscopist, observed that they were filled with crystals of what was later identified as urate, the salt of uric acid. In 1848, Alfred Baring Garrod in England reported excessive uric acid in the blood of gout patients, but not in persons with other types of arthritis. Garrod treated gout with lithium, which could dissolve the crystals, and speculated that it might be helpful in a variety of conditions, including mental disorders.

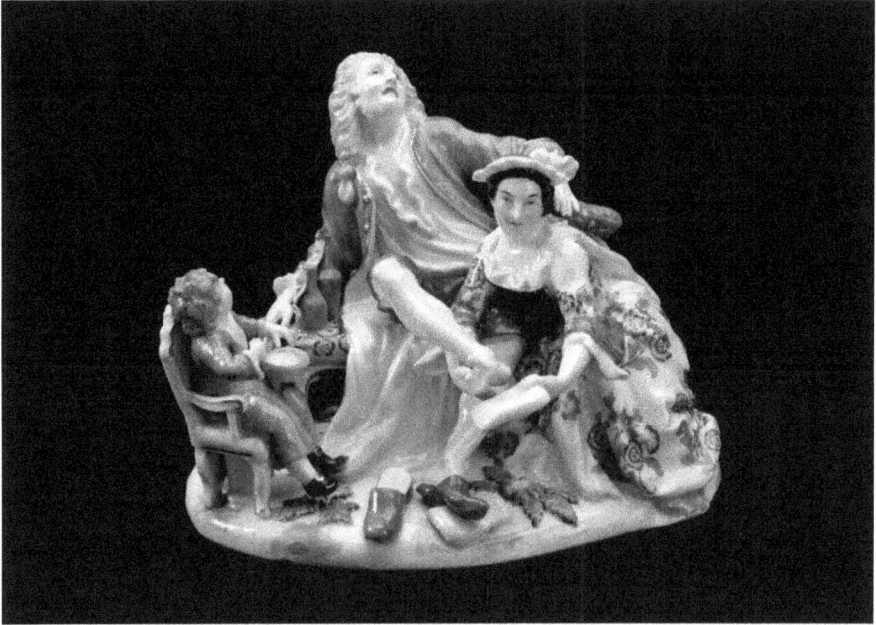

Figure 4-3: Porcelain figurine from Meissen, Germany, depicting a man with gout being comforted by his family. Gout is associated with excessive consumption of steak, liver, seafood, and alcohol, which historically led to it being thought of as an illness of the well-to-do, or 'the disease of kings.' It is more common in the overweight, and in older males.

In the late 19th and early 20th centuries, there was a growing idea that uric acid might be involved in a variety of other disorders, a so-called 'uric acid diathesis,' including 'brain gout.' Lithium had been used for some time to dissolve kidney and gall stones, and this history, coupled with Garrod's suggestion, led William A. Hammond (1829-1900), whom we mentioned earlier for his struggles against the wide use of a mercury-based drug in Union soldiers, to give it to his patients at Bellevue Hospital in New York.

In 1871, he reported the benefits of lithium bromide in treating mania. There was little interest at the time, and despite a large promising Danish study involving prevention of recurring depression, his observation languished for three quarters of a century, until it was re-discovered by Australian psychiatrist John Cade.

Cade served in World War II in Singapore, was captured by the Japanese, and was held in prison for three and a half years. As the only psychiatrist, he was put in charge of a small mental health unit. While there, he saw the effects of malnutrition, resulting in illnesses such as pellagra, in which lack of niacin (vitamin B_3) results in confusion, aggression, and dementia, and beriberi, in which thiamine (vitamin B_1) deficiency causes difficulty walking, pain, a form of amnesia, and confusion. In other situations, physical causes such as blood clots in the brain were found in patients with disturbed behavior. Traditional psychiatric teaching at the time emphasized problems in upbringing as the root of later psychiatric illness. These kinds of experiences, though, led Cade to think more about possible 'organic' causes of mental disorders. It is thought that he was impressed that some of his patients had fluctuating levels of mental clarity. Just as Frank Berger was thinking in 1945 about how anxiety would seem to come and go at different times (Chapter Three), Cade speculated about what the underlying physiology might be. It seemed to him that changes in mental processes might reflect the rise and fall of some toxic substance.

After the war, Cade returned to psychiatric work at a veteran's facility near Melbourne and set out to find the hypothetical toxic substance. He built a makeshift laboratory in an unused kitchen in the hospital. It was about as improbable a location for a revolutionary discovery in psychiatry as the surgical unit in the Bizerte Naval Hospital, where Henri Laborit began his work leading to the clinical discovery of chlorpromazine (Chapter Two). He began by injecting the urine of manic patients into guinea pigs and found that it made them substantially sicker than that from persons without mania. It turned out that the most toxic substance was urea, but he was puzzled because its amounts were similar in patients and non-manic persons. Something, he speculated, must be making the urea more harmful in manic patients, and he thought it might be uric acid. He planned to inject uric acid into the guinea pigs, but it is not very soluble in water, so he prepared it in the form of the soluble lithium urate. To his surprise, the lithium urate behaved the opposite of his prediction—it seemed to reduce the toxicity of urea. It turned out that this was produced by the lithium, which also made the animals quiescent.

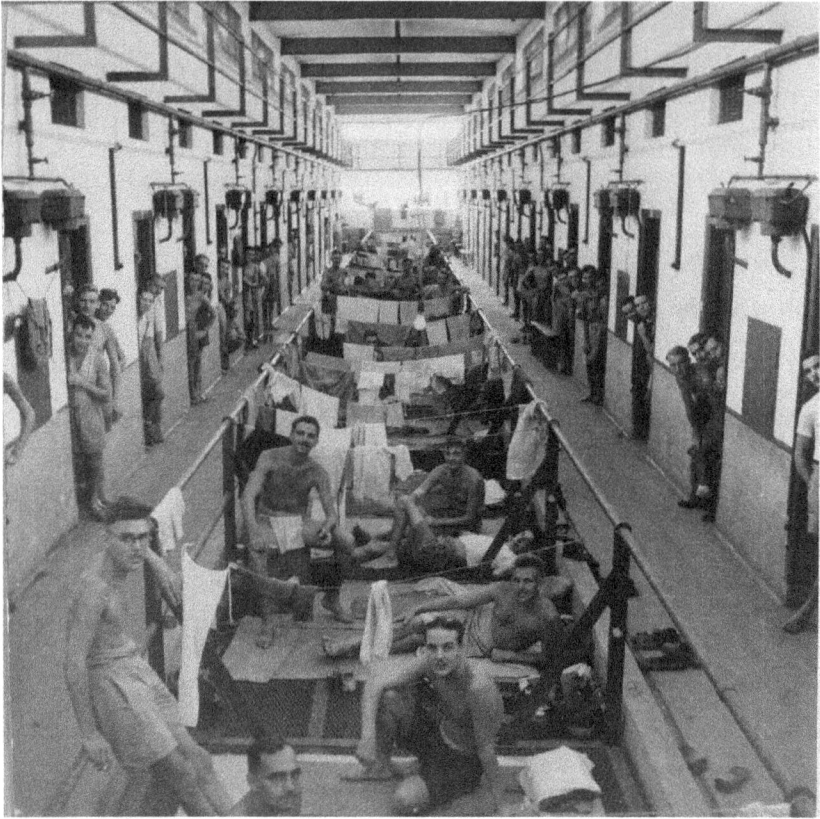

Figure 4-4: Allied troops shortly after being liberated from Changi prison in Singapore, where John Cade was held until September 1945. His experiences there may have influenced his growing belief that varying levels of toxic substances might influence the course of mental disorders.

Cade made the intuitive jump from seeing the animals made quieter to the notion that lithium might be useful in mania. After first giving himself some in an effort to determine the dose, he administered it to 10 manic patients and described very positive results in the medical journal of Australia in 1949. His report, like Hammond's so many years before, received very little interest. Cade followed up with uneventful studies with rubidium and cerium. He was also dispirited by the death of a patient, which was ascribed to lithium. Like Alexander Fleming, he went on to other things.

As it happened, lithium was in the news around the same time as Cade's discovery, for a very different reason. It had been in consumer products for other purposes—indeed, lithium citrate was an ingredient in the original 7 Up soft drink—but now lithium chloride was gaining popularity as a salt substitute. Sometimes it was taken in significant quantities, and reports began to appear of resultant toxicity and deaths. In 1949, the same year that Cade published his paper, the U.S. Food and Drug Administration took it off the market. Not surprisingly, the consequent worry about possible harmfulness made it very slow to be accepted as a medicine. In 1958, a blood test became available to determine therapeutic levels and lower the chance of toxicity. Even so, and despite the enthusiastic support of prominent psychiatrists in Europe and North America, it was only twenty years later in 1970 that it was approved in the U.S. for mania, and 1974 for prevention of recurrence of new episodes. Ultimately, this inorganic substance became one the first major advances, along with chlorpromazine, in modern psychiatry. It became so ubiquitous that at this point it is embedded in popular culture, with characters who receive it in movies as varied as *An Unmarried Woman* and *Stardust Memories*, and song titles such as Sting's 'Lithium Sunset' and Sirenia's 'Lithium and a Lover.' It is a good reminder in this history of evolving organic compounds which became modern drugs that nothing is simple, and inorganic substances have also played a role.

CHAPTER FIVE: METHYLENE BLUE AND OTHER DYES IN MODERN MEDICINE

In Chapter One, we dwelt on the role of methylene blue (MB) as an early treatment for malaria and as a precursor to other drugs such as chlorpromazine. We also mentioned that Paul Ehrlich and others had given it to psychotic patients, and that Ehrlich thought that it might have a role in psychiatry. It turns out that he was prescient in this, as in so many other matters. Almost 150 years after its creation as the first synthetic drug, it continues to have some medical uses, and it is being studied for potentially slowing down the progression of some types of dementia. Let's look at some of these:

Methylene blue in medical disorders

Methemoglobinemia and the 'blue Fugates' of Kentucky: Perhaps the best-known medical use of methylene blue is in a condition in which there is an excess of methemoglobin, a form of hemoglobin which does not carry oxygen. Normally it makes up only 1-2 percent of hemoglobin and is kept at this level by an enzyme which breaks it down, but in certain situations it can rise dramatically, producing a bluish-brown color to the blood, and blue skin in Caucasians. Symptoms can include shortness of breath, confusional states, myocardial infarction, seizures, or coma. Interestingly, one of the common causes is as a side effect of antimalarials and antibacterials including chloroquine and sulfonamides, as well as a variety of other drugs such as some local anesthetics and anticonvulsants

Methemoglobinemia can also have a genetic origin. A famous example was the 'blue men of Lurgan,' brothers from a town in Northern Ireland known for its history in the textile industry. They were seen by a Dr. James Deeny in 1942, treated with ascorbic acid and sodium bicarbonate, and their skin returned to normal in two weeks to a month.

Another well-known family descended from Martin Fugate, a French immigrant who settled in Troublesome Creek, Kentucky in 1820. Martin, whose skin had a bluish tint, married Elizabeth Smith, who was described as being 'as lovely as the mountain laurel.' They went on to have seven children, of whom four had blue skin. Though their abnormality was confined to their coloration and did not seem to affect their health, the Fugates were well known in the area and came to the attention of Dr. Madison Cawein, a hematologist at the University of Kentucky. In 1960, he and a nurse, Ruth Pendergrass, who had once seen such a person at the county health department, set off to find them. It was not so easy, as they were shy and sometimes when approached would flee. Ultimately, they connected with Fugate relatives Patrick and Rachel Ritchie. Cawein examined them, found that their blue color was not due to heart disease, and studied their blood samples. Luckily, he came across a paper describing such patients among the indigenous population from the Arctic Research Center in Anchorage, Alaska. It was determined that their coloration came from a recessive gene resulting in a functional loss of an enzyme ('NADH-cytochrome $b5$ reductase') which breaks down methemoglobin. This particular form of methemoglobinemia results in changes in color without inducing the ravages of the full-blown illness. Having an understanding of the chemistry involved and armed with experience with previous cases, Cawein chose to treat them with methylene blue dye. The Ritchies were skeptical, wondering how a blue dye could change their blue skin to pink, but agreed. He gave an injection of methylene blue and before his eyes over the next few minutes they changed color. This happy effect didn't last, as methylene blue is rapidly removed by the kidneys, but he sent them home with an ample supply of an oral preparation. As it turns out, the modern treatment for methemoglobinemia is oxygen plus an intravenous injection of methylene blue, after which improvement is often seen within an hour. After injection, methylene blue is converted by red blood cell enzymes into a colorless compound, which in turn converts methemoglobin into normal oxygen-carrying hemoglobin[*].

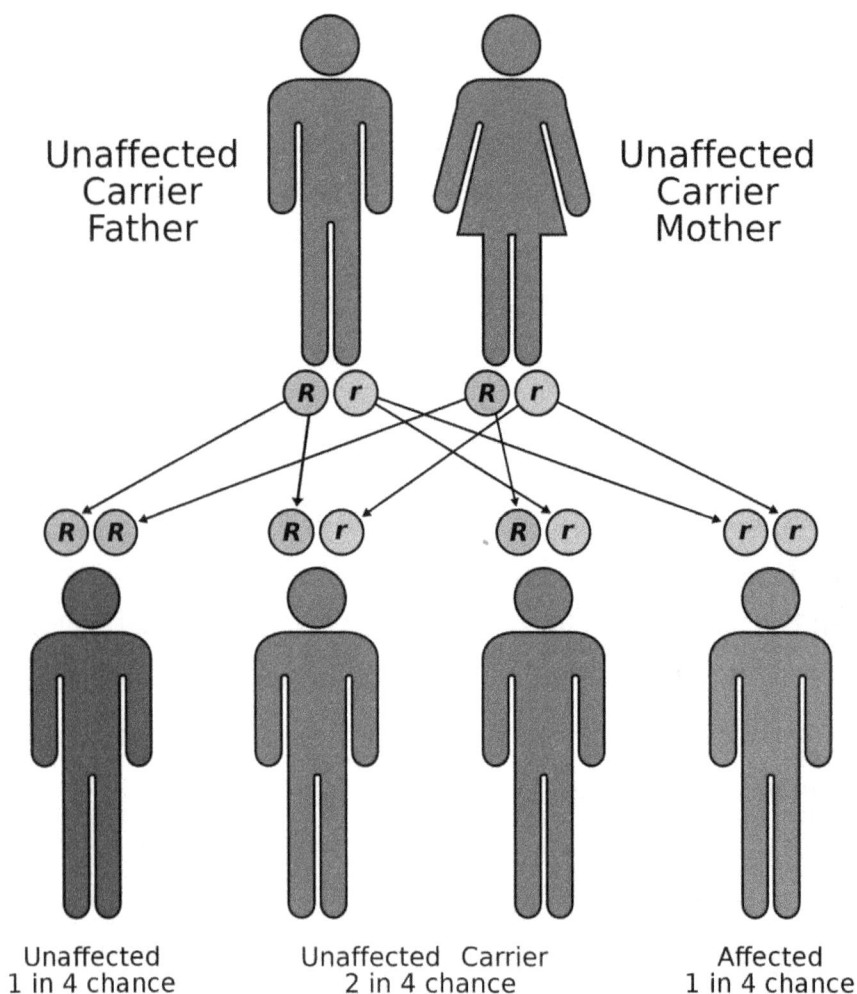

Unaffected
Carrier
Father

Unaffected
Carrier
Mother

Unaffected
1 in 4 chance

Unaffected Carrier
2 in 4 chance

Affected
1 in 4 chance

Figure 5-1: *In the most common form of inherited methemoglobinemia, the gene is recessive. As seen in this diagram, neither parent will have abnormal*

---

[*] Chemically, methylene blue does this by acting as an electron receptor in a process by which an enzyme converts the iron atoms in methemoglobin from the ferric (Fe^{3+}) to the ferrous (Fe^{2+}) state found in oxygen-carrying hemoglobin.

coloration, but if they carry the gene, one-quarter of their children are likely to have blue skin, but not necessarily other symptoms. In another, rarer, form of methemoglobinemia (not pictured here), one parent can transmit the gene, and the resulting illness can cause neurologic impairment and failure to thrive in infants.

As for the Fugates, now no longer blue, and with better transportation becoming available, they slowly spread out from the remote confined area in which they had traditionally lived and married into the general population in which this recessive gene was less common. The last known blue descendent was a baby born in 1975, a carrier whose coloration decreased with time.

Other medical uses of methylene blue: MB is used off-label to prevent or treat complications in the nervous system in patients who receive the anti-cancer medicine ifosfamide, which can cause psychosis, seizures, or coma. It is also used off-label to head off urinary tract infections in older persons, to treat priapism (painful prolonged erections induced by some drugs and other causes), and cyanide poisoning, and to help surgeons visualize certain kinds of tissues such as intestinal polyps or pre-cancerous growths. It has a role in disinfecting donated blood plasma. There has been renewed interest in once again using it for malaria, in combination with other drugs[17].

Methylene blue in psychiatry and neurology: Contemporary studies of methylene blue suggest that it is well-placed to be of benefit in some psychiatric disorders. Chemically, it can be considered a phenothiazinium or tricyclic phenothiazine[18], and indeed the same chemist, Heinrich August Bernthsen, who synthesized the phenothiazine molecule in 1883 had worked out the structure of methylene blue in 1885. It was, as we have seen, a historical precursor to the phenothiazine chlorpromazine and the tricyclic antidepressants (Chapter Two). It increases amounts of the neurotransmitters serotonin and norepinephrine in the brain*, as do many antidepressants. It also blocks activity of an enzyme known as nitric oxide synthetase, which is thought to be involved in depression. Older clinical studies have suggested that methylene blue may be beneficial for depression[19], and as adjunctive therapy in bipolar disorder[20] and schizophrenia[21]. It has been found to have an antidepressant-like effect in animal models of depression[22]. There is also some evidence from preclinical and clinical studies that it may have a role in slowing the progression of Alzheimer's disease[23,24,] possibly by reducing amounts of abnormally shaped 'tau protein,' which contributes to plaque formation in the brain[25]. Whether these treatments will come to any kind of clinical fruition is not clear, but it is interesting that almost 150 years after its discovery, methylene blue continues to be studied.

---

* Methylene blue inhibits MAO-A, and also promotes the release of serotonin and norepinephrine.

Other dyes in contemporary medicine

Traditionally, there has been a tendency to not use dyes in medicines, due to their causing color changes in tissues, but at the same time there has been increased interest in taking advantage of coloration, and in particular in light-sensitive substances. Molecules which change their shape in response to light are known as 'photochromic'; it is by this process, for instance, that sunglasses can be made which become darker when exposed to the sun. Indigo itself is not photochromic, but some derivatives, known as indigoid dyes, are. In effect, they and other photochromic dyes can be used as 'photoswitches,' which go far beyond novel color changes. Some have antibacterial or anti-cancer cell properties. They can also be incorporated into drugs, and then turn the drugs 'on' and 'off' in response to light. Indigoid dyes are also being explored for possible roles as organic semiconductors or in memory chips[26].

In 'photodynamic therapy,' a variety of dyes can attach to cancer cells and make them sensitive to light. For cancers on the skin, the dye may be applied directly, or for internal locations it is given intravenously. Laser lights are then shined on the newly photosensitive cancer cells, leading to their destruction.

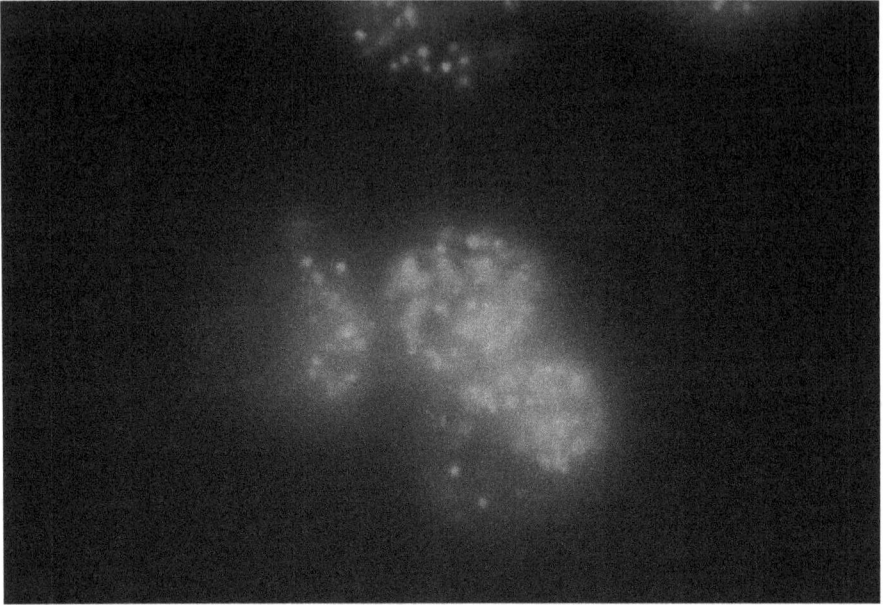

Figure 5-2: Photodynamic therapy: In this photo, cancer cells are absorbing the photosensitizing agent Photofrin (porfimer sodium). For cancer of the esophagus, for instance, Photofrin is given intravenously, and two days later, the tumor is illuminated by a laser.

Light-sensitive proteins can also be used in studying gene function. At any one time, only a small fraction of the roughly 20,000 genes in humans are activated, and normally they are turned on and off rapidly depending on the body's needs. In order to study this process, a technique known as optogenetics makes use of light-sensitive proteins from plants, which in nature provide the plant with information about day length. By combining these with other proteins which are capable of activating genes, researchers can target specific genes, and then shine lights on them, causing them to activate and hence provide information about their function[27].

Dyes, then, which were developed into drugs beginning in the 1800s, continue to have a role in medicine and science in the twenty-first century.

CHAPTER SIX: SUMMARY

Modern medicines in psychiatry were initiated by a series of discoveries in the 1950s and 1960s, often as a result of a combination of unexpected observations made by doctors or scientists who in turn were open to their possibilities and made intuitive leaps about new applications. Emblematic of this was Henri Laborit, who noticed that chlorpromazine, a new antihistamine he intended to use in surgery, produced in patients a kind of calmness and indifference that he thought might be useful in psychiatry; as a consequence, the first modern medicine for psychoses was born. Leading up to this and the many other discoveries of these decades, there was a century of birth and evolution of the process of making drugs. It began in 1856 with William Henry Perkin, a chemistry student who was looking to synthesize quinine, and instead ended up with a dark-colored sludge in his glassware, which he recognized might be useful as a fabric dye. It came into its own in 1858 when August Kekulé and Archibald Scott Couper independently demonstrated the immense possibilities that resulted from understanding the bonding properties of carbon atoms. The field of synthetic organic chemistry was born, making it possible to create a wide variety of compounds. Every builder, though, needs raw materials, and as a happenstance of history that was available too, in the cheap and abundant coal tar which was a byproduct of processing coal to produce coke for making iron and gas for lighting. These newfound chemical skills and plentiful raw material were turned to making fabric dyes initially, but over the years broadened into other areas including cosmetics, paints, food coloring, and medicines. One stimulus for medicines was the need to deal with malaria and sleeping sickness which were inhibiting imperial ambitions, and syphilis, which though less virulent than in past centuries, nonetheless was widespread and took a toll on the population. Not surprisingly, many of the medicines which appeared originated as dyes. Among these was methylene blue, springing from Paul Ehrlich's observation that it was toxic to malarial parasites, and which he recognized might be useful in psychiatry. Indeed, until World War I, the words 'dye' and 'drug' were often used synonymously.

In looking at the history of how medicines in psychiatry evolved, it became clear that it was not an isolated process. Rather, it involved an interaction with both infectious diseases and the medicines developed to treat them. Thus, a derivative of methylene blue, first a dye and then a drug, evolved into chlorpromazine, which was unsuccessfully tested as an antimalarial, but revolutionized the treatment of psychoses. The dye prontosil red became the first sulfa antibacterial agent; its discoverer found a derivative which was one of the building blocks for isoniazid, the precursor of iproniazid, the first MAO inhibitor antidepressant. Iproniazid itself was developed for tuberculosis, and its other possibilities were recognized because TB patients receiving it had improved mood, energy, and outlook. A search for a penicillin preservative led to meprobamate, which became the first modern tranquilizer. The examples go on and on, but in summary show a pattern in which the synthesis of drugs for infections and for mental disorders, through the grace of organic chemistry, were intertwined for many years. Even the illnesses themselves interacted: in 1917, malaria fever therapy was found to be beneficial for psychoses due to neurosyphilis and was tested less successfully for schizophrenia and bipolar disorder. Until the late 1940s, neurosyphilis contributed heavily to the populations in mental hospitals; with the advent of penicillin, there was a significant shift in the types of patients, and many psychiatrists turned their attention from the 'organic' to the 'functional' psychoses such as schizophrenia.

In the 1940s, the two fields, which had so fruitfully evolved together, began to separate. As we described earlier, antibiotics such as streptomycin and penicillin came from bacteria in soil and mold, and though synthetic means are also employed, today scientists primarily look for new antimicrobials by searching for products made by bacteria which are harmful to other bacteria. But the many years in which the fields were intertwined laid the foundations for the remarkable advances in psychiatric medicines in the next decades.

Much has been made of serendipity, the accidental quality of many of the discoveries in the 1950s and 1960s, and the same thing can be seen in this preceding period. Sometimes chance played a major role. In 1763, when the Reverend Stone tasted willow bark, he was spurred on when he noted that its bitter taste was similar to that of Cinchona bark used for malaria, leading him to pursue its possible medicinal qualities. Though it was a coincidence that the taste was much the same, and the connection with quinine was spurious, the powdered bark contained fever-reducing salicylic acid, later modified to become aspirin, one of the most widely taken medicines in the world.

More commonly, although the chance element was often there, it was usually in combination with recognition by a person who was willing to see something unusual and grasp its implications. No doubt any number of chemistry students might have ended up with dark-colored sludge in their glassware, but something about William Henry Perkin's background in painting and his sensitivity to color may have aided his recognition that his particular mess might become a fabric dye. Alexander Fleming's discovery of penicillin can be seen a number of ways. The story is usually told that one day he happened to notice that mold which had invaded a petri dish was destructive of bacteria, and he got the idea that it might become an antibiotic. Actually, Fleming was highly attuned to the idea that natural substances might be harnessed against infections in wounds. He had already discovered one antibacterial agent—lysozyme—and was looking for others. It is ironic that this same search blinded him to the full implications of penicillin treatment, initially limiting his vision to topical use in the wounds which he had thought about ever since World War I. Similarly, Frank Berger, who noticed that a penicillin preservative caused animals to become less active and made the leap that it might become a tranquilizer in humans, had been interested for some time in anxiety and how it comes and goes at different times. John Cade noticed that lithium produced quiescence in guinea pigs and made the intuitive leap that it might be useful in treating mania, but he did so in the context of looking for substances whose varying levels might be reflected in changes in mental status. Going back to the seventeenth century, Jesuit missionaries in the Eastern slopes of the Andes, seeing Indians using cinchona bark for non-malarial fevers and the chill from cold temperatures thought to try it for malaria, which may not have been endemic in the altitudes where they learned about the plant (Chapter Three). The intuition that led them to do this came from concern about the affliction in their lowland brothers. Usually the past experiences and interest of the discoverer, as well as a willingness to see and think about the unexpected, played as important a role as chance.

The two fields of developing drugs in microbiology and psychiatry are now far apart, and each faces its own challenges. Modern antibiotics derived from soil bacteria are becoming limited by the development of bacterial resistance, and new approaches are needed. Psychiatry moved on in the 1980s from the era of intuitive discoveries to one of rational design of drugs based on findings about the physiology of mental illness. It still faces the challenge of neurological and metabolic side effects of antipsychotics, as well as the search for agents which improve a broader range of symptoms in schizophrenia, and antidepressants which work by new mechanisms. Just as we couldn't foresee that methylene blue, discovered in 1876, is currently being looked at for use in Alzheimer's disease, and that other dyes play roles in cancer treatment and elucidating gene function, we don't know what will happen next. It would be fascinating to know how these times will be seen by a new historian looking back from some decades in the future.

Glossary

This glossary is provided for readers who would like to learn more about some of the more technical terms in the text.*

Alkaloids: Alkaloids are organic substances found in nature which include basic nitrogen atoms in their structure. They are produced by plants, fungi, and bacteria, and many have been made into medicines or recreational drugs. The main one mentioned In this book is the drug quinine, a treatment for malaria, derived from the bark of the cinchona tree. Other examples are morphine, caffeine, cocaine, as well as the hallucinogen LSD, derived from ergot, a fungus which grows on rye and other plants.

Antimicrobials, antibacterials, antibiotics: Antimicrobials refer to substances which kill or stop the growth of microorganisms, which include bacteria, viruses, fungi and parasites. Among these are external disinfectants such as bleach, used to clean non-biological

---

* Some of this explanatory material appears in the glossary of *THE CURIOUS HISTORY OF MEDICINES IN PSYCHIATRY* (see Selected Bibliography).

surfaces of a variety of organisms, and which should never be used on or in the human body. Other types of antimicrobials include antiseptics designed for topical use as antibacterial agents for wounds, and (the focus of this book) systemic medicines taken orally or by injection. The term *antibiotics* refers to antibacterial agents derived from organisms such as streptomycin and penicillin, but is also often more loosely applied to synthetically derived substances such as sulfonamides (which are technically non-antibiotic antibacterials). Agents which prevent the growth of bacteria are known as *bacteriostatic*, while those which kill them are known as *bactericidal*.

Histamine: A natural substance formed from the amino acid histidine, which plays a role in immune responses, gastric acid secretion, and blood vessel function, and acts as a neurotransmitter in the nervous system. Among its many effects are allowing white blood cells and proteins to pass through the walls of capillaries into tissues, dilating blood vessels, and lowering blood pressure. Chemically it is a monoamine, and thus in the same general family as serotonin, norepinephrine, and dopamine. In the nervous system, cells which communicate using histamine as a transmitter come from the posterior hypothalamus and spread out to influence wide parts of the cortex and other areas, where they tend to promote wakefulness. Its various functions are modulated by binding to receptors with four subtypes, named H1-H4.

Infectious diseases: Diseases caused by harmful organisms including bacteria, viruses, fungi and parasites. Malaria, for instance, is caused by an infection by the *Plasmodium* parasite, which is transmitted through the bite of the *Anopheles* mosquito. Yellow fever and COVID-19 are examples of viral infections.

Monoamine oxidase inhibitors and how they act: As described in Chapter Two, serotonin, norepinephrine, and dopamine are neurotransmitters which convey signals across the gap between neurons ('the synaptic cleft'). One of the ways in which the amount of monoamines available is regulated is by their chemical breakdown by a pair of enzymes known collectively as monoamine oxidase. One form of this enzyme, MAO-A, breaks down the monoamines serotonin, norepinephrine, melatonin, and epinephrine, while MAO-B breaks down other substances such as phenethylamine and benzylamine. Both process tyramine, dopamine, and tryptamine. Iproniazid blocks the actions of both enzymes, and its effect is irreversible. These qualities made it more prone to the 'cheese effect,' potentially dangerous hypertension resulting from eating foods containing the amine tyramine (which is also metabolized by MAO). Ultimately, safer MAOIs such as moclobemide that are selective for only MAO-A, and whose effects are reversible, became available. Moclobemide is marketed in the U.K., Canada, Australia, and other countries, though not in the U.S. Selegiline, which irreversibly blocks MAO-B, is used as a treatment for Parkinson's disease. The resultant increase in norepinephrine, serotonin and dopamine from blockage of MAO-A by iproniazid and later drugs, along with improvement in depressive symptoms, was one of the foundations of the monoamine hypothesis of depression (see next item).

Monoamine hypothesis of depression: This suggest that depression is a consequence of inadequate amounts of monoamine neurotransmitters. While foundational in the modern understanding of mood disorders, alternate views include the notion that there may be decreased activity of neurotrophic factors, which regulate generation of new cells and connections in the nervous system, and play a role in the response to new experiences. Endocrine changes in cortisol, thyroid and sex hormones have also been found. Low grade inflammation has been reported, and possible disorders of immune processes are being studied, as are genetic alterations of neurotransmitter function and the body clock regulation. These systems are inter-related. Many antidepressants, for instance increase amounts of monoamines, which in turn can alter both neurotrophic factors and hormonal processes. It is possible then, that some combination of these processes, or indeed others yet to be discovered, play a role in the genesis of mood disorders.

Neurotransmitters: Neurotransmitters are substances involved in the process of communication between individual nerve cells (neurons). In order to understand them, and how drugs affect their function, it's useful to look at how this communication is made possible. (A more detailed account can be found in the author's book *Understanding Antidepressants*, listed in the Bibliography.) The story begins with Santiago Ramon y Cajal (1852-1934), a Spanish pathologist whose microscopic studies led him to propose that neurons are not continuous but are able to signal each other at specialized conjunction points known as synapses. At these points the signaling neuron ('presynaptic') and the receiving neuron ('postsynaptic') are separated by a microscopic gap about 20-40 nM wide. Originally it was speculated that a signal crossing this gap might be electrical. In 1921, however, Otto Loewi (1873-1961), a German physiologist, studying frog's nerves, discovered chemical neurotransmission, in which substances known as neurotransmitters are released from the presynaptic neuron, and cross the gap between neurons to convey a signal. We now know that neurotransmitters attach ('bind') to specialized receiving points, known as receptors, which when stimulated alter the function of the receiving neuron. Although there are a handful of types of neurons communicating by traditionally electrical means, the vast majority of neuronal communication occurs by this chemical process. Among the neurotransmitters which appear important to psychiatric drugs were what became known as monoamines, substances such as serotonin, norepinephrine, and dopamine, which are involved in arousal, concentration, appetite, emotions, memory, and other processes.

It turned out, then, that the amounts of neurotransmitters available in the synapse would have profound effects on how neurons communicate. After they are released by presynaptic neurons, their amounts are regulated by several processes. Some of the transmitters diffuse out of the synapse into surrounding tissue. Other means include chemical breakdown by enzymes, and re-uptake back into the presynaptic cell by specialized structures known as transporters. Drugs can influence both the amount of transmitters released, as well as these types of processes. The MAO inhibitors, for instance, block enzymes which chemically break down monoamines, so that more remains available in the synapse. Others, such as the tricyclic antidepressants and SSRIs, act by interfering with the reuptake process, once again allowing more neurotransmitter to accumulate.

Organic chemistry: The study of organic compounds, containing carbon atoms bound to carbon or other atoms in a special manner known as covalent bonding, which involves the sharing of electron pairs. These include hydrocarbons (carbon plus hydrogen), but also others including oxygen, sulfur or nitrogen. A related class, organometallics, are, as the name indicates, molecules which include organic components in combination with metals such as mercury, nickel or zinc.

Psychopharmacology: Psychopharmacology has been defined in several ways, including the study of drugs for mental illness, or the effects of drugs on specific processes including thinking, sensation, and mood. Some have emphasized the distinction from psychopharmacotherapy, the observation of the effects of drugs in a clinical setting, from psychopharmacology, which is based on organized scientific procedure. The word 'psychopharmakon' may have first been used in 1548 by Reinhardus Lorichius, a German theologian, in a book of prayers, in which it seems to refer to the healing power of prayer for dealing with adversities. In the twentieth century, it appeared in a medical context several times in the 1920s and 1930s, but became generally accepted after an influential paper by that title in 1960, when it also began to appear in the Index Medicus a bibliographic database of medical journal articles.

Rational drug design: An approach to developing new drugs based on using the principles of synthetic organic chemistry to manipulate molecules, with a goal derived from a biological theory of the origins of mental disorders and information on biological drug targets. The development of selective serotonin reuptake inhibitors (SSRIs) in the 1980s is an example of this process.

Receptors: As we mentioned in the section on neurotransmitters, these substances attach to specialized parts of the synapses known as receptors as a crucial step in communicating between neurons.

Although drugs can produce their effects by a number of means, probably the most important is binding to these same sites, which, when activated, produce changes in the functioning of the neuron. Receptors have several qualities which are important. One of these is specificity, that is, they will only respond when a substance with a very precise structure attaches to them. Another is that drugs may differ in the stickiness ('affinity') with which they attach, which in addition to the number of receptors, contributes to the amount of drug required to cause a change in cell function. Receptors may also have a number of subtypes, which produce different effects when stimulated. Finally, the structure of many receptors located on the cell surface may extend through the membrane and in effect form a kind of communication from the outside to the inside of the cell. Particularly important are receptors of this type which are regulatory proteins, which may act by various mechanisms. Some, such as the receptor for benzodiazepines located on the $GABA_A$ receptor, include a channel between the outside and inside of the cells, and when stimulated allow ions to pass through, quieting the cell and making it less likely that it will generate a signal to other neurons. Another kind, when stimulated, releases regulatory substances inside the cell, which in turn influence how the cell functions. An example of this are 'G protein-coupled receptors,' which include, for instance, receptors for serotonin. Various forms of this type of receptor are the targets of up to 30 percent of currently used medicines.

Receptor agonists: Drugs which, when binding to a receptor, stimulate its function. Other drugs which bind to receptors and block its function are known as antagonists. Some compounds bind to receptors and cause it to produce an effect opposite to that produced by agonists and are known as 'inverse agonists.'

Sleeping sickness: An illness of sub-Saharan Africa caused by protozoan parasites in the genus *Trypanosoma*, which are transmitted primarily by the bite of infected tsetse flies. It has two major forms, and the one caused by *Trypanosoma brucei gambiense* is the most common. Typically the illness has two stages, first involving fevers, swollen lymph glands and joint pains one to three weeks after infection, and a second stage usually weeks or months later which can include nervous system symptoms such as confusional states, personality changes, and alterations in body rhythms. Medications such as fexinidazole and others are available for treatment.

Synapses: See 'Neurotransmitters'

Tricyclic antidepressants, SSRIs, and how they act: As we described in the Glossary section for monoamine oxidase inhibitors, there are several mechanisms by which neurotransmitters are removed from the synaptic cleft, and MAOIs act by one of them, by inhibiting an enzyme which breaks them down. Another method by which neurotransmitters are removed is by reuptake into the presynaptic neuron by specialized sites known as transporters. Tricyclic antidepressants work by blocking these transporters, so that there is an increase in the amount of the monoamine neurotransmitters remaining in the synaptic space. Various tricyclics differ in the degree to which they differentially affect serotonin or norepinephrine. Their action is not limited to blocking reuptake, however. They also act as antagonists at one of the types of serotonin receptors known as 5-HT$_2$, which may also result in antidepressant properties. Additionally, they act as antagonists at some receptors for other neurotransmitters such as histamine and acetylcholine, which results in some of their side effects. When a later generation of antidepressants, the selective serotonin reuptake inhibitors became available in the 1980s, one of their perceived benefits over the tricyclics was that their major action was indeed 'selective,' that is, confined to blocking serotonin reuptake.

Trypanosomiasis: see 'Sleeping sickness'

Uric acid and mania: Although it is easy to dismiss the quaint nineteenth century notion of 'brain gout,' it turns out that John Cade's 1949 observations about uric acid in the urine of manic patients continues to be of interest. Studies in recent years have found increased levels of serum uric acid in persons with first episode mania. Uric acid is formed from the chemical breakdown of substances known as purines, and one of the many aspects of gout can involve more rapid processing of these substances. Some writers have speculated that the more rapid removal of the purine adenosine, which has a number of actions in the nervous system including sedation or promoting sleep, could theoretically lead to some of the symptoms of mania. Further readings on this include: S.S. Chatterjee et al.: Serum uric acid levels in first episode mania, effect on clinical presentation and treatment response: Data from a case control study. Asian J. Psychiat. 35: 15-17, 2018. https://www.ncbi.nlm.nih.gov/pubmed/29723720 and Scientific American: A new target for treating mania? SA Mind 27, 6, 11 (November 2016) doi:10.1038/scientificamericanmind1116-11

Yellow fever: A disease now largely found in South America and Africa, due to a virus, and transmitted by the bite of *Aedes* or *Haemagogus* mosquitos. Its symptoms can vary from a relatively mild condition with fever and aches to severe illness damaging the liver with the resulting yellow skin of jaundice, as well as bleeding and shock. Symptoms often appear within three to six days of infection. Persons who recover tend to have immunity from future episodes. A vaccine has been available since the late 1930s.

Of interest in this book: in 1793 there was a severe yellow fever epidemic in Philadelphia, which led to the deaths of as many as 5000 of the city's 50,000 inhabitants. It was thought to be due to infected mosquitoes brought on ships of French refugees from what is now Haiti, who had emigrated after leaving behind a slave revolution at the time.

Selected Bibliography

American Chemical Society: Discovery and development of penicillin. Accessed April 23, 2020.

https://www.acs.org/content/acs/en/education/whatischemistry/landmarks/flemingpenicillin.html

Campbell, W.C.: Serendipity and new drugs for infectious disease. ILAR Journal 46: 352-356, 2005. https://doi.org/10.1093/ilar.46.4.352

Chakraborty, S. and Rhee, K.Y.: Tuberculosis drug development: history and evolution of the mechanism-based paradigm. Cold Spring Harb Perspect Med. 2015 Apr 15;5(8):a021147. doi: 10.1101/cshperspect.a021147. Accessed April 23, 2020.

Howland, R.H.: Methylene blue: the long and winding road from stain to brain: Part 2. J. Psychosoc. Nurs. Ment. Health Serv. 54: 21-26, 2016.   DOI: 10.3928/02793695-20160920-04

Mendelson, W.B.: *Understanding Antidepressants*, Independently published, 2018. Available on Amazon. https://www.amazon.com/Understanding-Antidepressants-Wallace-B-Mendelson-ebook/dp/B07B4GWKSN/ref=sr_1_1?keywords=understanding+antidepressants&qid=1575918156&s=digital-text&sr=1-1

Mendelson, W.B.: *Understanding Sleeping Pills*, Independently published, 2019. Available on Amazon. https://www.amazon.com/Understanding-Sleeping-Pills-Wallace-Mendelson-ebook/dp/B07FSY24PY/ref=sr_1_1?keywords=understanding+sleeping+pills&qid=1575918240&s=digital-text&sr=1-1

Mendelson, W.B: *The Curious History of Medicines in Psychiatry*, Pythagoras Press, New York, 2020. https://lnkd.in/gR9sg3h

World Health Organization: Guidelines for the treatment of malaria. Third Edition. World Health Organization, 2015. https://books.google.com/books/about/Guidelines_for_the_Treatment_of_Malaria.html?id=IVo0DgAAQBAJ

Picture Credits

The author's assessment is that all images are in the public domain or presented under the terms of Section 107 of the U.S. Copyright Law (the 'Fair Use' provision). When appropriate, all reasonable efforts have been employed to trace copyright holders and to get their permission for the use of copyright material. The author apologizes for any errors or omissions in this list and will gratefully include any corrections in future editions if notified.

Cover: 1882 New Zealand two pence postage stamp depicting Queen Victoria, in mauve color, from Wikimedia Commons. According to the New Zealand Crown Copyright Act of 1994, images of New Zealand stamps are in the public domain '50 years after issue for stamps issued before 31 December, 1944.'

Figure P-1: The great exhibition of 1862. Archives of Bayer AG, from Wikimedia Commons: 'This work is free and may be used by anyone for any purpose.'

Figure P-2: Hercules and the discovery of the secret of purple. Peter Paul Rubens, from the Musee Bonnat-Helleu, from Wikimedia Commons: 'This work is in the public domain in its country of origin and other countries and areas where the copyright term is the author's life plus 100 years or fewer.'

Figure P-3: Kekule's drawing of the structure of benzene. August Kekulé, from Wikimedia Commons: 'This work is in the public domain in its country of origin and other countries and areas where the copyright term is the author's life plus 70 years or fewer.'

Figure P-4: West German stamp commemorating the centenary of the discovery of benzene. From Nightflyer, from Wikimedia Commons: 'This image of a simple structural formula is ineligible for copyright and therefore in the public domain, because it consists entirely of information that is common property and contains no original authorship.'

Figure P-5: Ouroboros statue. Kulttuurinavigaattori, from Wikimedia Commons: 'This work is free and may be used by anyone for any purpose.'

Figure 1-1: Gasworks. From A.J.F. Maenen, from Wikimedia Commons: 'This work is in the public domain in its country of origin and other countries and areas where the copyright term is the author's life plus 70 years or fewer.'

Figure 1-2: Methylene blue in ethanol. From Lecaimant, from Wikimedia Commons: 'This file is licensed under the Creative Commons Attribution-Share Alike 3.0 unported license.'

Figure 1-3: Microscopic images of bacteria. From Frederick Treves (1853-1923), in the Francis A. Countway Library of Medicine. Digitized by Open Knowledge Commons and Harvard Medical School, from Wikimedia Commons. This is in the public domain as its first publication was prior to January 1, 1925.

Figure 1-4: Chipping Norton. From Robert Powell, in Wikimedia Commons: 'This file is licensed under the Creative Commons Attribution-Share Alike Unported License.'

Figure 1-5: Aspirin bottle, 1899. Archives of Bayer AG, from Wikimedia Commons: 'This work is free and may be used by anyone for any purpose.'

Figure 1-6: The Great Phenol Plot. New York World, from Wikimedia Commons: 'This media a file is in the public domain in the United States. This applies to US. Works where the copyright has expired, often because its first publication occurred prior to January 1, 1925, and if not then due to lack of notice or renewal.'

Figure 3-2: Cinchona officinalis. Hermann Adolf Koehler, from Wikimedia Commons: 'This work is in the public domain in its country of origin and other countries and areas where the copyright term is the author's life plus 100 years or fewer.'

Figure 3-3: Returning from the Orient. Benjamin Rabler, from the Wellcome Collection. In the public domain, under Attribution 4.0 International (CC BY 4.0) license.

Figure 3-4: Advertisement for quinine. Arthur Rothstein, from Wikimedia Commons: 'This work is in the public domain in the United States because it is a work prepared by an officer or employee of the United States Government as part of that person's official duties under the terms of Title 17, Chapter 1, Section 105 of the U.S. Code.'

Figure 3-5: Al Capone. World Wide Photos, Chicago Bureau (Federal Bureau of Investigation), from Wikimedia Commons: 'This image or file is a work of a Federal Bureau of Investigation employee, taken or made as part of that person's official duties. As a work of the U.S. federal government, the image is in the public domain in the United States.'

Figure 3-6: *Penicillium.* A.C.J. Corda, 1838. From Wikimedia Commons: 'This work is in the public domain in the United States because it was published (or registered with the U.S. Copyright Office) before January 1, 1925.'

Figure 3-7: An American Penicillin poster. Science History Institute, from Wikimedia Commons: 'This file was provided to Wikimedia Commons by the Science History Institute as part of a cooperation project.... This work is in the public domain in the United States because it is a work prepared by an officer or employee of the United States Government as part of that person's official duties under the terms of Title 17, Chapter 1, Section 105 of the U.S. Code.'

Figure 3-8: Cultures of *Streptomyces.* G. Terry Sharrer, National Museum of American History, from Wikimedia Commons: 'This image was released by the National Cancer Institute, an agency part of the National Institutes of Health, with the ID 1827.... This image is in the public domain and can be freely reused.'

Figure 4-1: Cinnabar. James St. John, from Wikimedia Commons: 'This file is licensed under the Creative Commons Attribution 2.0 Generic license.'

Figure 4-**2:** Decorative jar for mercury pills. Wellcome Collection. In the public domain, Attribution 4.0 International (CC BY 4.0) license.

Figure 4-**3:** Porcelain figurine from Meissen, Germany. Wellcome Collection. In the public domain, licensed under Attribution 4.0 International (CC BY 4.0) license.

Figure 4-**4:** Allied troops shortly after being liberated from Changi prison. State Library of Victoria Collections, from Wikimedia Commons: 'This image is of Australian origin and is now in the public domain because its term of copyright has expired.'

Figure 5-**1:** Methemoglobinemia chart. Cburnett, from Wikimedia Commons: 'This file is licensed under the Creative Commons Attribution-Share Alike 3.0 Unported license.'

Figure 5-**2:** Photodynamic therapy. National Cancer Institute, from Wikimedia Commons: 'This image is in the public domain and can be freely reused.'

References

[1] Mendelson, W.B.: THE CURIOUS HISTORY OF MEDICINES IN PSYCHIATRY, Pythagoras Press, New York, 2020.

[2] Muller, O. et al.: How worthwhile is methylene blue as a treatment of malaria? Expert. Review of anti-infective therapy 17: 471-473, 2019.
https://www.tandfonline.com/doi/full/10.1080/14787210.2019.1634545

[3] Bodoni, P.: Dell'azione sedativa del bleu di metilene in varie forme di psicosi. Clin. Med. Ital. 21: 217-222, 1899. Ehrlich, P. and Leppmann, A.: Uber schmerzstillende wirkung des methylenblau. Dtsch. Med. Wochenschr. 16: 493-494, 1890.

[4] Mendelson, W.B.: *THE CURIOUS HISTORY OF MEDICINES IN PSYCHIATRY* by Wallace B. Mendelson, Pythagoras Press, New York, 2020.

[5] Murray JF: A century of tuberculosis. Am. J. Resp. Critical Care Med. 169: 1181-1186, 2004. https://doi.org/10.1164/rccm.200402-140OE

[6] Gerhard Domagk – Biographical. NobelPrize.org. Nobel Media AB 2020. Sun. 12 Apr 2020. <https://www.nobelprize.org/prizes/medicine/1939/domagk/biographical/>

[7] Paisseau, G.: Malaria during the war. Lancet, 193: 749-751, 1919. DOI:https://doi.org/10.1016/S0140-6736(00)95225-5

[8] Jenkins, R. et al.: Malaria and mental disorder: an population study in an area endemic for malaria in Kenya. World Psychiatry 16(3): 324–325, 2017. doi: 10.1002/wps.20473

[9] Mendelson, W.B.: The psychiatric effects of COVID-19 treatment: we need to be aware of the potential consequences of chloroquine on mental health. Psychology Today, March 31, 2020. https://www.psychologytoday.com/us/blog/psychiatry-history/202003/psychiatric-effects-covid-19-treatment

[10] Telgt, D.S. et al.: Serious psychiatric symptoms after chloroquine treatment following experimental malaria infection. Ann. Pharmacother. 39: 551-554, 2005. DOI: 10.1345/aph.1E409

[11] Cintas, P.: How serendipity led to an early treatment. Nature 419, 431 (2002). DOI https://doi.org/10.1038/419431b

[12] R. Bodker et al.: Relationship between altitude and intensity of malaria transmission in the Usambara mountains, Tanzania. J. Med. Entomology 40: 706-717, 2003.
https://www.researchgate.net/publication/9028222_Relationship_Between_Altitude_and_Intensity_of_Malaria_Transmission_in_the_Usambara_Mountains_Tanzania

[13] WHO: Disease Information: International Travel and Health.
https://www.who.int/ith/diseases/malaria/en/

[14] R.L. Nevin and A.M. Croft: Psychiatric effects of malaria and anti-malarial drugs: historical and modern perspectives. Malar. J. 15: 332, 2016. https://doi.org/10.1186/s12936-016-1391-6

[15] Garavito, G. et al.: The in vivo antimalarial activity of methylene blue combined with pyrimethamine, chloroquine and quinine. Mem. Inst. Oswaldo Cruz 107: 820-823, 2012.
https://pubmed.ncbi.nlm.nih.gov/22990975/https://pubmed.ncbi.nlm.nih.gov/22990975/

[16] E.P. Abraham: Fleming's discovery. Rev. Infectious Dis. 2: 140, 1980. https://academic.oup.com/cid/article-abstract/2/1/140/336691?redirectedFrom=PDF

[17] O. Muller et al.: How worthwhile is methylene blue as a treatment for malaria? Expert Rev. Anti-infective Therapy. 17: 471-473, 2019. DOI: 10.1080/14787210.2019.1634545

[18] M. Wainwright and L. Amaral.: The phenothiazinium chromophore and the evolution of antimalarial drugs. Trop. Med. Int. Health 10:501-511, 2005.

[19] G.J. Naylor, A.H.W. Smith and P. Connelly: A controlled trial of methylene blue in severe depressive illness. Biol. Psychiat. 22: 657-659, 1987. https://doi.org/10.1016/0006-3223(87)90194-6

[20] M. Alda et al.: Methylene blue treatment for residual symptoms of bipolar disorder: Randomised crossover study. Brit. J. Psychiat. 210: 54-60, 2017. DOI: https://doi.org/10.1192/bjp.bp.115.173930

[21] S.I. Deutsch et al.: Methylene blue adjuvant therapy of schizophrenia. Clin. Neuropharm. 20: 357-363, 1997. https://jhu.pure.elsevier.com/en/publications/methylene-blue-adjuvant-therapy-of-schizophrenia-3

[22] B.H. Harvey et al.: Role of Monoamine Oxidase, Nitric Oxide Synthase and Regional Brain Monoamines in the Antidepressant-Like Effects of Methylene Blue and Selected Structural Analogues.

Biochem. Pharmacol. 80: 1580-1591, 2010. DOI: 10.1016/j.bcp.2010.07.037

[23] M. Oz, D.E. Lorke, and G.A. Petrolanu: Methylene blue and Alzheimer's disease. Biochem. Pharmacol. 78: 927-932, 2009. DOI: 10.1016/j.bcp.2009.04.034

[24] R.H. Howland: Methylene Blue: the long and winding road from stain to brain. J. Psychosoc. Nurs. Ment. Health Serv. 54: 21-26, 2016 DOI: 10.3928/02793695-20160920-04

[25] J. Schartner et al.: An ATR-FTIR Sensor Unraveling the Drug Intervention of Methylene Blue, Congo Red, and Berberine on Human Tau and Aβ. ACS Med. Chem. Lett. 8: 710-714, 2017. DOI: 10.1021/acsmedchemlett.7b00079

[26] T. Heine et al.: Indigoid dyes by group E monooxygenases: mechanism and biocatalysis. Biol. Chem. 400: 939-950, 2019. DOI: https://doi.org/10.1515/hsz-2019-0109

[27] L.R. Polstein and C.A. Gersbach. A light-inducible CRISPR-Cas9 system for control of endogenous gene activation. Nature Chem. Biol. *11: 198-200*, 2015; DOI: 10.1038/nchembio.1753

www.ingramcontent.com/pod-product-compliance
Lightning Source LLC
Chambersburg PA
CBHW060036210326
41520CB00009B/1148